Vaccines: The Past, COVID-19, and the Future

Vaccines: The Past, COVID-19, and the Future

Written by: Mohathir Sheikh, Fariha Khan, Angela Kazmierczak, & Yemariam Abebayehu

Edited by: Alyssa Kulchisky, Austin Mardon, & Catherine Mardon

Designed by: Josh Kramer

Published by Golden Meteorite Press
2021

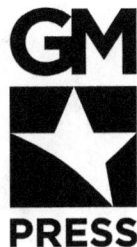

GM
PRESS

First Printing: 2021

ISBN: 978-1-77369-598-3

Golden Meteorite Press
103 11919 82 St NW
Edmonton, AB T5B 2W3
www.goldenmeteoritepress.com
aamardon@yahoo.ca
Alberta, Canada

Table of Contents

Preface

From immunology experts at VBI Vaccines (2016), the future developers of the prophylactic hepatitis b vaccine:

> Since their earliest and most rudimentary introduction, vaccines have fundamentally changed the way modern medicine is practiced and have eliminated or managed the incidence of some of the most devastating human diseases ... The path to discovering effective vaccines was long and difficult. The work required a number of brave research pioneers and clinicians (para. 1).

Chapter 1: Vaccine History

The Pre-Vaccine Era and the Eventual Creation of Vaccines

John Heywood once wrote that where there's smoke, there's fire (Ammer, 2013). It's also fair to say that where there's a vaccine, there's an outbreak. Like smoke and fire, vaccines and outbreaks go hand-in-hand. Since the World Health Organization (WHO) declared COVID-19 a pandemic in 2020, our interactions have revolved around preventive measures. As early as March 11th, officials and doctors have pleaded we wash our hands, wear our masks, distance feet apart, and, finally, get vaccinated (WHO, 2020). We're here to discuss that last suggestion, "to get vaccinated."

Now we wouldn't ever claim that this book will transform your life or move you to tears, but it just might save it. That counts for something and makes reading it worthwhile. From this book, you will gain a scientific understanding of how vaccines work and how moments from the past, COVID-19, and the future all net together. But, to understand the significance, the thought process behind making vaccines, and the nuances in-between, we must study the world's first recorded outbreak of a disease and how the long-negated germ theory furthered vaccine developments. To begin, we'll start with the smallpox endemic and its origins as it pegs when vaccine history all began.

Unbeknownst at the time, smallpox would become

humanity's first of many viral diseases we would develop a vaccine for. In fact, smallpox has inflicted over three hundred million deaths since 1900, only beshrewing its final blow in the United States in the 1950s (American Museum of Natural History, 2021). The majority of countries and age groups (the elderly, adults, and especially children) would suffer from the oozing, pus-filled pustules. That is, of course, until a vaccine was developed, but that didn't occur overnight or even after a matter of months. Only after centuries of trial and error, would the disease be declared officially eradicated by the World Health Organization in the 1980s—truly a major marker as humanity's first virus to be eliminated worldwide. Before progressing any further, though, let's explore the events that catalyzed the development of vaccines and of what inoculation consisted of in its earliest forms.

The Origins of Smallpox
Though several scientific discoveries and breakthroughs have emerged since World War II and in the 21st century, the origins of smallpox remain unknown. Historians' earliest, most credible recordings of smallpox date to 3,000 year-old skin lesions on the mummy of Ancient Egypt's former king, Ramses V (Geddes, 2006). King Ramses V, who reigned from 1150-45 BCE, is rumoured to be one of the first persons to contract smallpox (Tikkanen, 2021). It is believed it was a breakthrough from Egypt's agricultural irrigation system that bred smallpox in Egypt's land and India's water (Geddes, 2006). While a controlled watering system expedited the country's food stockpile, population size, travelling, and trading routes in ways once inconceivable, for the next two thousand years the virus continued transmitting as an endemic, an illness "native to a particular people" (Geddes, 2006; Merriam-Webster, 2021, p. 1). On average, 3 out of

every 10 people died from smallpox, and survivors were left scathed in severe scarring from scabs (Centers for Disease Control and Prevention (CDCP), 2021).

Smallpox and Its Forms

Smallpox, a word of Latin origin, means "spotted" (Gilman, 2018). Its name comes from the raised bumps (or pustules) surfacing on top of the skin of the face or body. The disease is an infectious and sometimes fatal variola virus consisting of two forms, one is called by scientists major smallpox and the other variola is called minor (Food and Drug Administration (FDA), 2018). As it was severely contagious, only dairymaids and smallpox survivors nursed those who were sick, as they exhibited immunity to the virus (Riedel, 2005).

Major Smallpox

Major smallpox, the most lethal and common of the two, consists of four types: "ordinary (the most frequently caught); modified (mild and occurring in vaccinated persons); flat; and hemorrhagic" (FDA, 2018, para. 1). Major forms of smallpox hold a mortality rate of 30% and often lead to one's demise if "a hemorrhagic [or a flat] form of the disease develops" (FDA, 2018, para. 1; Geddes, 2006). To ancient civilization's relief, incidences of hemorrhagic and flat seldom occur. Hemorrhagic strains are known for causing fatality because of their brief incubation period, which is the time between contraction and exhibiting symptoms. Its short incubation period results in doctors not recognizing it quickly, and, in addition to its dangers, the vaccine fails to ward against it (FDA, 2018).

Variola Minor

A variola minor form of the disease (also known as variola

alastrim), is uncommon and less noxious as its mortality rate is only 1% or less (FDA, 2018). According to Strauss and Strauss (2008), "variola minor was endemic in Africa and the Americas and coexisted with variola major" ("Eradication of Smallpox").

If a person was to develop variola minor, he or she generally exhibited the weakened symptoms of major smallpox including a less extensive rash, less scarring, and a mild, short-lived fever (UPMC Center for Health Security, 2014). Despite its weakened symptoms, variola minor is still highly contagious and spreads via respiratory droplets and through direct contact with scabs (CDCP, 2021).

Before and After Incubation
An airborne disease means that sneezing, coughing, sharing bedding or clothing, or coming into contact with bodily fluids deduces infection. Upon infection, the virus enters the body via the respiratory tract. Once incubation has completed, which takes 7 to 19 days in ordinary and modified cases, it is shortly followed by a boiling fever, head and body aches, vomiting, rashes spreading from the tongue and mouth to the face and feet, pustular sores, and scabs that fall off. The virus is most contagious when the sores fill with a "thick, opaque fluid [that] have a dent in the center" (CDCP, 2021, para. 3).

The Countries Facing an Endemic
Old medical writings and Sanskrit texts (which are North Indian monumental scripts) confirm the transmission of smallpox in countries beyond Ancient Egyptian and Indian borders (CDCP, 2021; Cardona, n.d.). Around the 4th century Common Era (CE), early Chinese writings described a rash-like disease emerging in theirs and neighbouring countries. From historians' analysis of trading routes and writings, Japan

and China had transferred the disease to Korea after bartering goods (CDCP, 2021). Soon after the Arab expansion of the 7th century, India wrote akin descriptions but ascribed it to the Hindu god of smallpox, Sitala Mala (Geddes, 2006). Then, in the 10th century, Asia Minor recorded similar descriptions. Travelling, extended trading routes, and increased population sizes are often pinpointed as the causes for transmission (CDCP, 2021).

In the early 1500s, "European exploration and colonization introduced the disease to the Caribbean and mainland Americas" (Geddes, 2006, para. 10). Progressing into the 16th century, smallpox was the primary cause of death in Europe, India, China, and southwestern Asia. The curse of smallpox, inflicting the loss of millions of people, stirred doctors, farmers, and even royals to find the antidote.

Controlling Smallpox Through Variolation
Depending on which source you read, variolation originates from either China or India (Boylston, 2012).
To minimize the blow of smallpox, China and India practiced the early forms of inoculation by variolation in the 1500s. The word variolation, which does not translate "to vaccinate," comes from the minor form of smallpox, the variola virus (CDCP, 2021).

Variolation, sometimes resulting in a healthy person's demise, entailed scratching minor variola pustules into the arm or inhaling pox sores into the nose to develop an immunity or foothold over the disease. Subjects would then develop two smallpox symptoms, fever and widespread rashes. Many countries noted over time that fewer died after undergoing variolation, but not every country, group, or doctor approved of it, despite it being the insertion of a minor form (CDCP, 2021).

Lady Mary Wortley Montagu

Lady Mary Wortley Montagu (1689-1762), who was a noble and a scarred survivor of smallpox, introduced variolation to the "United Kingdom from Turkey in 1721" (Stewart & Devlin, 2005, para. 4). Montagu, from 1721-22, began advocating for the practice after a diplomatic trip to Turkey. Her husband, Edward Montagu, appointed Ambassador to the Ottoman Empire, granted Lady Montagu access to harems, the lady's living quarters in Turkey (Gearon, n.d.). That is where Montagu learned of variolation, which was said to keep the women's complexion smooth and scar-free. After contracting smallpox as a child and being left unrecognizable from facial scars, Lady Montagu hurried to have her children inoculated (Stewart & Devlin, 2005).

With variolation now growing in popularity in England by 1721, some religious groups and most doctors opposed the act, deeming it unsafe, demoralizing, or demonic—an act of murder being performed on children (Stewart & Devlin, 2005). Variolation was already routinely practiced by the Chinese, Turks, and Africans. That same year, after an African slave named Onesimus shared the story of his variolation during childhood, the act spread throughout America. South America soon learned of it in 1728. To outside countries, inoculation was a means to build immunity, to survive, and to avoid extreme scarring.

While many of the English were morally troubled or frightened about inserting a pustule into the skin, according to Geddes (2006), "the then Princess of Wales, Caroline of Ansbach, had her children inoculated, which led to the procedure of variolation becoming fashionable in England" (para. 22). According to Stewart & Devlin (2005), "quantitative studies performed in 1722 in London, England and 1726 in Boston, Massachusetts showed mortality rates were reduced from 1 in 6 in non-variolated patients to as low as 1 in 50 in variolated patients" (para. 5). In fact, upon refining the variolation technique, numbers reduced to 1 in 500.

Lady Montagu was willing to suffer hostility and physical violence for her beliefs in variolation. Montagu is celebrated today for "introduc[ing] smallpox inoculation to Britain and Western Europe" (Gearon, n.d., para. 1). Variolation continued in England until superseded by vaccination in 1798. In 1842, the English parliament ruled variolation a felony (Encyclopaedia Britannica, n.d).

Clinical Trial Pioneer, Dr. William Watson
Dr. William Watson (1717-1787), electricity collaborator and ally of Benjamin Franklin, was a physician at the Hospital for the Maintenance and Education of Exposed and Deserted Children, more commonly known as the Foundling Hospital, in 1762 (Encyclopaedia Britannica, n.d.). While there, preventing a smallpox outbreak in the dorm rooms was Dr. Watson's focus. As recorded in the 18th century, 80% of deaths befell from smallpox infection in children 5 years-old or less (Geddes, 2006).

In 1767, Dr. Watson performed one of the first clinical trials (Stewart & Devlin, 2005). In this trial, he studied variolation samples at differing times of maturity and of various preparation techniques. Dr. Watson's first question of study surrounded the age of pock samples (the inoculum) and if it affected an inoculation's efficacy. Inoculum use at the time was sporadic and varied from doctor to doctor—some physicians administered early lesions and mature pocks, while others did old, resolved lesions (Boylston, 2014). His second question surrounded patients' pre-treatment. Most doctors recommended patients consume a meatless diet and purgatives "to expel matter from the stomach and bowels" (Boylston, 2014, para. 7). Many doctors also prescribed Hermann Boerhaave's popular antimony and mercury concoction as a pre-treatment to inoculation, as they theorized it cured the 'variolous poison' causing smallpox. But Dr. Watson doubted a poisonous substance, such as mercury, would have any efficacy or benefits in consuming. Rather than expressing his doubts about the use of mercury to other practitioners, as he would likely face ridicule, Dr. Watson chose to prove its ineffectiveness through trials (Stewart & Devlin, 2005).

On went Dr. Watson, inoculating several boys and girls at the same time and of similar ages and genders. In his findings, he discovered "pre-treatment with laxatives without mercury was sufficient, [and] that use of fluid from an active smallpox lesion was optimal" (Stewart & Devlin, 2006, p. 330). Not only did he refine the pox inoculation, but Dr. Watson became the first doctor to implement study design, control groups, and quantitative analysis in the field of medicine.

The Father of Vaccines, Edward Jenner
Dr. Edward Jenner (1749-1823), an English surgeon and lover of nature, "underwent variolation as a boy and would recall with horror his experiences in isolation with post-vaccination

fevers" (Stewart & Devlin, 2006, p. 330). Apprenticing under a nearby surgeon after completing grammar school at the age of 13, Dr. Jenner, at 21, was later mentored by Dr. John Hunter, one of the lead surgeons in London. Dr. John Hunter, his teacher and loyal friend, asked him: "Why think [i.e., speculate]—why not try the experiment?" (King, 2021, para. 4). Harkening to Dr. Hunter's words of knowledge in his practice, in 1796 Jenner experimented with the belief that dairymaids never succumbed to the blinding and disfiguring smallpox if infected by cowpox first (Riedel, 2005).

Cowpox, also known as vaccinia, is typically a mild disease that transfers to humans from milking cattle with ulcerated teats. Vaccinia closely identifies with the variola virus, "the causative virus of smallpox," and the names are sometimes used interchangeably (Tikkanen, n.d., para. 1).

Signs and Symptoms of Cowpox
Infected individuals typically suffered pustule-sores on the hands and face, but they at times experienced generalized symptoms, including: tiredness, fever, vomiting, sore throat, enlarged lymph nodes, and conjunctivitis or swelling in the eyes (Ngan, 2008). More prevalent in the 1800s, it is uncommon for a dairy worker or for any person to contract cowpox in the 21st century. Today's industrial farming methods, specifically automatic milking through robots, minimizes a dairy worker's handling and pulling of the teats, which is the point of cowpox transference (Ryall, 2018).

In Ryall's (2018) BBC interview with Dr. Robert Smith, the clinical lead scientist at Public Health Wales, he reported, "a total of 29 laboratory reports of cowpox were received by the public health laboratories (PHLS) communicable disease surveillance centre between 1975 and 1992" (para. 24). This reveals how few cowpox cases have emerged since the farming industry's technological advances and upticks in sanitary practices. While ten or fifteen years more years may pass before a doctor encounters cowpox again, it does happen, though seldom.

To further supplement our understanding of the lowering numbers of cowpox, according to Tikkanen (n.d.), "during the 1980s, researchers discovered that rodents were also a natural reservoir for the virus and that rodents, not cattle, were responsible for most cowpox infections in humans" (para. 2). Robotic and sanitary practices of today lessen the frequency of cowpox, a zoonotic disease, transmitting from animal to person, albeit, other outbreaks still arise from mismanaging animals, mishandling incidents, and unorthodox animal farming (Illinois Office of the Vice-Chancellor for Research & Innovation; Dalton, 2021).

It is common practice in the majority of the world, in at least 74% of countries to be exact, for people to be prompted to wear gloves or to wash his or her hands when handling rats or birds (World Health Organization, 2019). Most people altogether avoid handling animals, unless for research purposes, farming, or for keeping animals as domestic pets. Still, Ebola, the 1918 Spanish flu, and H5N1 bird flu are all attributed to wild eating (Dalton, 2021). Virologists and doctors continue to be on guard for cowpox or any other outbreaks.

The Logistics of Dr. Jenner's Cowpox Trial
To begin his test, on May 14th, 1796, Dr. Jenner extracted a fresh cowpox specimen from the hand of a dairymaid, named

Sarah Nelmes, and inoculated the lesion into an 8 year-old boy, James Phipps (King, 2021). The young lad, Phipps, developed a mild fever, "discomfort in the axillae," shivers, and a loss of appetite, but on the 10th day, he restored to good health (Riedel, 2005, p. 24). Now able to progress further into testing, in July of 1796, Dr. Jenner inoculated smallpox into Phipps and no signs of smallpox developed. That confirmed the dairymaids' cowpox tale.

In the following year, in 1796, Dr. Jenner submitted his findings to the Royal Society only to have his study rejected. In response, by 1798, Dr. Jenner administered cowpox to several more participants, recording its effectiveness in a tiny booklet, consisting of three parts, titled, "An Inquiry into the Causes and Effects of the Variolae Vaccinae, a disease discovered in some of the western counties of England, particularly Gloucestershire and Known by the Name of Cow Pox" (Riedel, 2005, p. 24). As you may have guessed, the English abhorred his sentiments and the medical community was divided (King, 2021; Riedel, 2005).

The Vaccination
A more important point of his study for our discussion here is that one of the sections in Dr. Jenner's booklet, the first, named his newest procedure vaccination. To disseminate the word, in Latin, vacca means cow, and cowpox translates to vaccinia (Riedel, 2005). When combining the Latin words it forms Dr. Jenner's to-be coined term: "vaccination". Over time, vaccine, meaning the cowpox inoculation, became applied loosely and to other inoculums (Merriam-Webster, n.d.).

Having published a three-part book series, Dr. Jenner returned to London to find recipients to inoculate but for three months no one dared volunteer—a by-product of the medical community's rejection for his booklets. However, Londoners willed for a cowpox dose via other physicians, eventually making the inoculation grossly popular and credited as the official method of smallpox prevention (Riedel, 2005).

Surgeon Dr. Henry Cline was the first to help popularize the inoculum, after Dr. Jenner shared some samples with him. Then, in 1799, Drs. George Pearson and William Woodville encouraged the vaccination to patients (Riedel, 2005). While the doctors furthered the agenda of the vaccine, "Dr. Pearson tried to take credit away from Jenner, and Dr. Woodville, a physician in a smallpox hospital, contaminated the cowpox matter with smallpox virus" (King, 2021, para. 9). To put it frankly, the doctors undermined his vaccine and bred confusion during the pinnacle of a preventive breakthrough. But, unrelenting in proving his findings to remaining skeptics, Dr. Jenner resolved he'd perform a nationwide survey to confirm his findings and to refine the procedure (Riedel, 2005). Hiccups, chicanery, and deaths occurring along the way, the survey, yet again and through many trials, confirmed his hypothesis.

Confident of its ability to prevent smallpox, Dr. Jenner promoted his smallpox vaccine more feverously, and "the procedure spread rapidly to America and the rest of Europe and soon was carried around the world" (King, 2021, para. 9).

Distributing the Cowpox Vaccine
Now that England had acquired the antidote, the conflict of distributing to other regions and countries surfaced. Unfortunately, inoculating the arm of a single patient was

laborious and necessitated a considerable amount of time from a doctor. Kean (2021) details the strenuous inoculation process:

> People with cowpox developed blister-like sores filled with a fluid called lymph. Doctors would prick open the sores, smear the lymph on silk threads or lint, and let it dry. They would head to the next town over and mix the crusty lymph with water to reconstitute it. Then they'd scratch the fluid into the arms or legs of people there to give them cowpox. (para. 6)

As explained by Kean, vaccinating Londoners was time-consuming but manageable. However, doctors would face greater difficulties when travelling two hundred and fifteen miles to their neighbour, Paris, France. As doctors would realize, the lymph lost its potency and verged expiry. That made distributing to Western countries, including the United States and Canada, an impossible feat. It was only by chance that a ship containing usable cowpox samples docked in Newfoundland in 1800. Chance was not a long-term solution though, and physicians had to think of how they'd distribute it to far away countries riddled with smallpox.

The solution to ensure that fresh inoculum arrived in Western countries, in 1803 health officials had 22 Spanish orphans boarded onto The Royal Philanthropic Vaccine Expedition and, throughout their travels, the doctors infected them with cowpox in pairs of two (Kean, 2021). After nine to ten days, another round of boys were infected. Planning for the last two boys to ripen fresh cowpox lesions upon their arrival to America, in March of 1804 doctors would hurry to extract the material from a single sore left on a boy's arm for inoculation.

Considering the era, the 1800s, the orphans, ages 3 to 9, likely never consented to boarding the ship and becoming carriers of cowpox, but fortunately, Spanish king, Carlos IV, promised hearty amounts of food, free education, and new adoptive parents for their sacrifices (Kean, 2021). In the end, King Carlos IV honoured those promises, and the children found homes in Mexico.

Dr. Jenner is Officially Credited Developer of the Smallpox Vaccine

In 1802, a year before the orphans set sail, the value of Dr. Jenner's inoculation was finally acknowledged by the British Parliament in England (Riedel, 2005). Earning worldwide recognition and accolades, Dr. Jenner did not seek wealth or any self-gain through his discovery. For his many personal sacrifices, dedication to refining and sharing his antidote, and success in saving millions of lives, the government awarded him £10,000 in 1802. Five years later, it was topped off by an additional £20,000. In 1823, at his cottage while sitting in his dimly lit study room, Dr. Jenner died of a massive stroke. In the 1980s, smallpox would be declared indefinitely eradicated.

Vaccine Pioneer, Louis Pasteur

Louis Pasteur (1822-1895), a painter, and later microbiologist and chemist, was regarded as an average student throughout his early education, yet he exhibited impeccable drawing and painting skills (Ullmann, n.d.). First painting canvases for museums across France, Pasteur later obtained an Arts degree, a Science degree, and a doctorate. He then researched and taught for several years at Dijon Lycée before transferring to the University of Strasbourg in 1848. The following year, in 1849, Pasteur engrossed himself in resolving an issue with tartaric acid (Biography.com, 2021).

Tartaric acid is "a colourless or white odourless crystalline acid" detected in many fruits and fermented wines, and it is often incorporated as a food additive in baking powders, soft drinks, and in tanning and photography (Collins English Dictionary, n.d., para. 1). The acid is a "water-soluble dicarboxylic acid existing in four stereoisomeric forms, the commonest being the dextrorotatory (d-) compound found in fruits" (Collins English Dictionary, n.d., para. 1).

Upon studying paratartaric acid by passing light through it, Pasteur discovered the crystalline shared a similar composition to tartaric acid. Hypothesizing the acids had akin compounds but different structures, Pasteur observed the crystallites under a microscope to confirm. At closer inspection, the crystals were of different types, albeit mirroring each other (commonly known today as molecular asymmetry). In conclusion, he found that studying composition was "not enough to understand how a chemical behaves. The structure and shape [were] also important" (Biography.com Editors, 2021, para. 4). This catalyzed the beginning of the field of stereochemistry.

Following Pasteur's ground-breaking discovery in chemical behaviour, he was promoted to professor of chemistry and dean of the science faculty at the University of Lille in 1854 (Biography Editors, 2021). While there, he aimed to resolve issues with manufacturing alcoholic beverages, as they always soured during travels. Conducting various tests and recording his observances, Pasteur contributed his findings to Joseph Lister's and Robert Koch's germ theory of disease. After releasing his findings, Pasteur convinced most of Europe, a once major skeptic, of the truth in the germ theory.

To remedy a solution for the spoiling drinks, Pasteur invented the process—which is also named after him—pasteurization. The act of pasteurizing substances, which is still practiced today, involves heating and cooling a liquid to kill off any bacteria (Biography.com Editors, 2021). Revolutionizing the manufacturing industry, Pasteur had demonstrated how organisms, such as bacteria, were the agents souring wine, milk, and beer. But that's not all Pasteur discovered about germs, as we will see later.

What Is the Germ Theory?
According to Biology Dictionary Editors (2017), the germ theory of disease, which scientists are still unfolding, is discussed as the following:

The germ theory of disease is based on the concept that many diseases are caused by infections with microorganisms, typically only visualized under high magnification. Such microorganisms can consist of bacterial, viral, fungal, or protist species. Although the growth and productive replication of microorganisms are the cause of disease, environmental and genetic factors may predispose a host or influence the severity of the infection. (para. 1)

As Pasteur had discovered, it was a particular bacteria causing issues in preservation. In conclusion, Pasteur saw validity in Lister's and Koch's germ theory, specifically in how bacteria may invade the body or a host of other things. However, what enabled these organisms to spread was beyond the researchers' understanding.

Additionally, Lister, Koch, and Pasteur failed to grasp the importance of basic sanitation, including washing hands before treating patients, sanitizing surgery frocks coats, and wearing face protection while surgically operating (Augustyn, n.d.). Not until 1847 Dr. Ignaz Semmelweis, a Hungarian-Jewish doctor beyond his time, discovered how basic sanitation stopped the spread of infection (Flynn, 2020).

To add to his misery, Dr. Semmelweis, the pioneer of handwashing, was doubted years after his death until "advances in the field of antiseptics" (Flynn, 2020, para. 27). Though Dr. Semmelweis hadn't fully realized the extent of his discovery, he identified an organic bacteria on the hands of doctors that was causing unnecessary deaths at a maternity ward. In the 1900s, Dr. Semmelweis' findings were heavily praised and birthed the favourite catchphrase of health officials, who often say it while uncontrollably salivating: "wash your hands" (Markel, 2015).

Pasteur's Application of the Germ Theory Leads to Vaccine Developments

Rescuing the silk industry in 1865 by preventing contamination from microbes, Pasteur, a man of many accomplishments, accidentally discovered the first vaccine for the chicken cholera disease. He had exposed chickens to the "attenuated form of a culture," and decided to observe how the birds, over several generations, exhibited increasing resistance to cholera (Biography.com Editors, 2021, para. 8).

Mindful of how attenuated cultures stimulated immunity in the chickens, which was an extension of the germ theory, Pasteur developed vaccines for the diseases, including, cholera, tuberculosis, anthrax, and smallpox. Then, in 1882, Pasteur attempted developing a rabies inoculation. To test his modified culture, Pasteur inoculated his fortunate subject, Joseph Meister. Meister, a 9 year-old boy, was suffering after a bite from a rabies-infected dog (Biography.com Editors, 2021). Pasteur's rabies vaccine demonstrating efficacy, he rose to fame and was credited "France's highest decoration, the Legion of Honour" (Biography.com Editors, 2021; Ullmann, n.d., para. 2). Unfortunately, now with sanitary practices upheld to a higher standard in surgeries and during childbearing, the poliovirus made an erupt, unexpected entrance in countries over the globe (The CPP, 2021).

The History of Poliovirus
The poliovirus, one of the first severe diseases to plague human civilization, has inflicted humanity since 1400 BCE (The College of Physicians of Philadelphia, 2021). Polio, short for poliomyelitis, is one of three types of poliovirus. All three forms are members of the Enterovirus genus.

According to WHO (2021), "50% of polio cases occur in children under the age of three" (para. 1). Polio is known for targeting children, but many adults have also contracted the disease. Roughly 98% of polio cases are mild and no symptoms develop, but as for 1-2% of severe cases, throat and chest paralysis or death often occur. In paralytic polio, temporary or permanent paralysis develops once the virus enters the bloodstream and attacks the nerve cells (The CPP, 2021).

To date, the largest outbreak of polio happened in the 1990s in countries with relatively high standards of living, notably in the United States (The CPP, 2021). During this time, while many other diseases were reduced by epic proportions from sanitation measures and widespread vaccination, polio kicked into overdrive, infecting countless children.

Higher standards in sanitation were linked to the soaring numbers of polio (The CPP, 2021). As ascertained by scientists, proper sanitation in maternity wards had delayed when a child contracted the disease. But delays in contraction required the child's system to fight the host on its own, as his or her immune system was no longer protected by maternal antibodies. Before changes in sanitation, infants, in the first months of life, originally caught polio through contaminated water supplies and effortlessly fought off the minor form from maternal protection.

The 1955 Polio Vaccine
With major outbreaks of polio occurring since 1894 in America, adults and mainly children suffered from the virus. In the 1900s, one of those unfortunate adults to contract polio was future American President, Franklin D. Roosevelt. Recovered but partially paralyzed, Roosevelt became "instrumental in raising funds for polio-related research and the treatment of polio patients" (History.com Editors, 2021, para. 2). Eventually Dr. Jonas Salk, in 1948, would receive a grant to study polio and to formulate a polio vaccine.

Dr. Jonas Salk Appoints the Polio Vaccine
Dr. Jonas Salk, an American virologist and medical researcher, was head of the research laboratory at the University of Pittsburgh in 1947. Awarded the task of creating a polio vaccine, Dr. Salk prepared an early version of the vaccine by 1950. The process included killing "several strains of the [polio]virus and then inject[ing] the benign viruses into a

healthy person's bloodstream. The person's immune system would then create antibodies designed to resist future exposure to poliomyelitis" (History.com Editors, 2021, para. 3).

A problem soon arose, though. Dr. Salk's obtaining of such large quantities of the poliovirus was never attempted before and his only other option—the use of live strands— was deemed risky, as it could spread polio in the bodies of those inoculated. It led Dr. Salk to contemplate using monkeys to grow the virus. Not long after, fortunately, to Dr. Salk's advantage, "in 1949 John Enders, Thomas Weller, and Fredrick Robbins discovered that poliovirus could be grown in laboratory tissue cultures of non-nerve tissue" (Science History Institute (SHI), 2021, para. 6). Borrowing from the virologists' discovery, Dr. Salk no longer acquired tribes of monkeys to harvest viruses.

Instead, Dr. Salk's procedure for "growing large quantities of the three types of polioviruses" included growing cultures on monkeys' kidney cells (SHI, 2021, para. 7). Afterwards, he followed by killing the viruses with formaldehyde. Once injected, the monkeys were protected against paralytic poliomyelitis. In 1952, Dr. Salk began testing the vaccine on children who had naturally contracted polio. Measuring the children's antibody levels before vaccination, Dr. Salk was pleased to note increased antibody levels post-vaccination (SHI, 2021). After running additional clinical tests and demonstrating its efficacy, Dr. Salk's vaccine became available to Americans in April of 1955 (History.com Editors, 2021).

Albert Sabin's 1962 Oral Polio Vaccine
After vaccine production errors left 200 American children

paralyzed and thousands sick of polio, the production of Salk's inoculation ebbed. Health officials were encouraged, however, that reported cases of polio in 1957 decreased to under 6,000—a record low (History.com Editors, 2021).

To encourage Americans to continue vaccinating, in 1962, Albert Bruce Sabin, a Polish-American medical researcher, released an orally-taken polio vaccine to replace Dr. Salk's jab (Science History Institute, 2017). During the time Dr. Salk had begun conducting trials for his vaccine, many scientists, including Sabin, experimented with attenuated live-virus vaccines. The reason being, scientists hypothesized only a live-virus provided lasting immunity to polio. Additionally, Sabin thought a tablet was superior, safer to administer than injections.

In Sabin's experiment, he grew many "virus strains in animals and tissue cultures and eventually found three mutant strains of the virus that appeared to stimulate antibody production without causing paralysis" (Science History Institute, 2017, para. 15). Once he found testing successful, he inoculated himself, his family, prisoners from Chillicothe Penitentiary, and fellow research associates.

Now presenting his inoculation to producers, Sabin failed to find support because of Salk's already successful polio vaccine (Science History Institute, 2017). But, once Sabin successfully inoculated the Russians, those at the time members of the Soviet Union, the pharmaceutical company Pfizer finally agreed to produce the live-vaccine and to perfect its production technique in British facilities in the 1950s. The live-virus, often delivered in drop-form or on top of a sugar cube, eventually replaced Salk's vaccine, becoming the official polio vaccine for years to come. In 1994, WHO declared polio eradicated because of mass immunization campaigns in Central and South America.

Prevention and Control of Polio

As discussed earlier, both adults and children contracted polio. In fact, anyone not immune to the poliovirus can become infected. Individuals susceptible to polio include those not vaccinated, who have not been fully vaccinated, or improperly vaccinated (e.g. missing a scheduled shot). Half of the polio cases (50%) occurred in children and infants as they were not immune to the virus (WHO, 2018). Today, pregnant mothers and carriers and those with weakened immune systems still run at a higher risk of contracting polio (Johnson, 2018). Thus, to prevent future outbreaks and to develop an immunity to severe diseases, oral polio vaccine (OPV) and now inactivated poliomyelitis vaccine (IPV) shots, amongst other vaccines, are administered to infants. While polio is not a threat in Canada or the United States anymore, some countries still struggle with outbreaks, including Pakistan, Afghanistan, and Nigeria (Government of Canada, 2018). Health officials recommend that before travelling to these countries or any outside countries, travellers should receive a booster or the vaccines necessitating that location, as "different countries have different health risks and may require specific vaccines" (Tellado, 2019, "Do My Kids Need Vaccines?").

Generally speaking, infants and children hold a greater risk of "vaccine-preventable diseases because their immune systems are less mature and less able to fight off infection" (Public Health Association of BC, 2021, para. 2). From contracting any vaccine-preventable diseases, it can be dangerous and life-threatening for everyone. Vaccinating children at the appointed times—often starting as early as two months of age—protects them the best and as early as possible (Public Health Association of BC, 2021). Most vaccines administered today are live, attenuated viruses—an inoculation consisting of a germ or weak form of the disease (VBI Vaccines, 2016, para. 11). It is important to also note that while Sabin and Dr. Salk developed the polio vaccines, yet another disease emerged, largely impacting Americans: measles.

The History of Measles
In the 9th Century, a Persian doctor published the first written account on measles. Fast forward, in 1757, a Scottish physician, Francis Home, "demonstrated that measles is caused by an infectious agent in the blood of patients" (CDCP, 2020, para. 2). Then, not long ago, in 1912, an average of 6,000 deaths and an estimated 3 to 4 million Americans contracted the disease every year. That's until a vaccine was developed in 1963 (CDCP, 2020). More recently, and despite a cost-effective vaccine being available, in 2018, a total of 140,000 deaths—mostly consisting of children—resulted from measles (WHO, 2019).

Measles, an airborne virus of the paramyxovirus family and one of the most contagious diseases in the world, spreads through direct contact and the air (WHO, 2019). Infected persons typically experience a high fever, runny nose, coughing, watery eyes, white spots inside the cheeks, and rashes on the upper neck and face. When severe forms of the virus develop, blindness, encephalitis (brain swelling), diarrhoea, pneumonia, dehydration, and ear infections follow.

Dr. Thomas Peebles, Developer of the First Laboratory Vaccine for Measles

In 1954, Dr. Thomas Chalmers Peebles (1921-2010), a recent graduate from Harvard Medical School, was tasked by Dr. John Enders, the finder of tissue cultures for polio and the Nobel Prize winner of 1954, to develop a measles vaccine (Martin, 2018; The CCP, 2010). Dr. Peebles agreed, working alongside Dr. Enders in his laboratory at Boston Children's Hospital (The CCP, 2010).

Once being notified of an outbreak at a private school in Boston, Dr. Peebles, who was determined in his studies of the virus, quickened to isolate the measles virus. Hurrying to obtain permission from the school's principal, Dr. Peebles collected "blood samples from each of the sick boys" and swabbed the children's throats (The CPP, 2010, para. 2). As Dr. Peebles had hoped for, in February of 1954, he identified David Edmonston's sample as containing measles virus-laden blood. Overlooking the significance of the blood sample, Dr. Enders transferred Dr. Pebbles to another department. Little did Dr. Enders realize at the time that the sample (commonly referred to as the Edmonston sample) would be used for preparing future measles, mumps, and rubella (MMR) vaccines (Martin, 2018).

Parting ways, Dr. Peebles continued harvesting generations of the measles virus and inoculating monkeys with the disease. In the meantime, Dr. Enders went on to develop the measles vaccine, using the original blood sample taken by Dr. Peebles. As Martin (2018) suggests, "that first tissue sample from David Edmonton has almost eradicated the disease in most developed countries. Dr. Peebles' identification of the virus was the necessary first step" (para. 9).

Dr. Peebles later studied the tetanus vaccine and discovered that booster shots only needed to be administered once every ten years, not every year (Martin, 2018). His finding, which is of great value, reduced the risk of experiencing any potential, unnecessary side-effects.

The Father of Modern Vaccines, Maurice Hilleman

"This guy, whatever he touched, he developed a vaccine out of it. We owe him an incredible, incredible debt... The company [Merck Vaccine Division] currently produces seven vaccines, all developed by Maurice Hilleman." (Adel Mahmoud, 2005, as cited in Dove, 2005, p. 52)

A discussion on modern vaccines would be sorely lacking if it failed to mention Maurice Hilleman. Maurice Ralph Hilleman (1919-2005), a microbiologist and avid vaccine developer, innovated many areas of the sciences, including, virology, immunology, cancer research, epidemiology, and vaccine development (Tulchinsky, 2018). Hilleman, often known as "the man behind childhood immunizations," would invent more than 40 vaccines in his six decades working at Merck & Company (Tulchinsky, 2018, p. 443; Dove, 2005).

Hilleman's Background Story

Hilleman was raised on his uncle's homestead in Miles City, Montanna. His family moved to the farm after the tragic loss of his mother two days after his birth. Maurice was one of eight children his father cared for. At the farm, the family suffered from poverty, routinely enduring grimy, unsanitary conditions (Tulchinsky, 2018).

Amid the Great Depression in 1937 and now a young man, Hilleman graduated from high school (Tulchinsky, 2018).

He was later accepted to Montana State University and won a full scholarship—in fact, several throughout his academic studies. At the age of 21 and although still living in unpleasant conditions, Hilleman double-majored in chemistry and microbiology. Not long after, in 1944, he received a Ph.D. following his award-winning dissertation on chlamydia.

Upon graduation, Hilleman received several offers in the field of academia, but he decided on working in the pharmaceutical industry. Landing himself a research position at E.R. Squibb & Sons, Hilleman immersed himself in developing vaccines. As mentioned earlier, "producing vaccines requires introducing a weakened live or dead agent—i.e., virus, bacteria, parasite, or another infective organism, or part of the organism—that can stimulate the production of antibodies" (Tulchinsky, 2018, p. 444). In consideration of American troops "at the Pacific front in Japan" that urgently needed immunization, Hilleman first focused on developing the Japanese B encephalitis vaccine.

Modern Influenza Vaccines
After his success, in 1948, Hilleman became chief of the Department of Respiratory Diseases at Walter Reed Army Medical Center (Tulchinsky, 2018, p. 445). He was tasked with studying respiratory illnesses of military significance and with devising a strategy for influenza prevention.

As defined by Merriam-Webster (2021), influenza is "an acute, highly contagious, respiratory disease caused by any of three orthomyxoviruses: influenza A, influenza B, and influenza C" (paras. 1-4). From his study, Hilleman "demonstrated that influenza A viruses underwent gradual and progressive minor antigenic characteristics (an immune response) called 'drift and shift,' which are the basis of modern influenza vaccine strategies" (Olanski & Lancet, 2005, as cited in Tulchinsky, 2018, p. 445). Duda (2020) further explains the characteristics of drift and shift:

Influenza strains are constantly mutating. A small change to the genetic makeup of influenza strains is referred to as antigenic drift, while a major change is called antigenic shift. While these designations are mainly relevant to scientists, they help explain why you can contract the flu more than once and why the influenza vaccine is changed annually (and may be less effective in some seasons than others). (para. 1)

Although not stated by Duda, drift and shift is one of Hilleman's several findings that transformed our approach to modern vaccines. Drift and shift not only describes the characteristics of influenza, but it explains why a multitude of vaccines and flu shots are developed in our modern world.

Some of the other vaccines credited to Hilleman includes Hong Kong flu (1957), measles (1963), mumps (1967), Hong Kong flu pandemic (1968), rubella (1969), MMR (1969), meningococcal polysaccharide (1974), pneumococcal pneumonia (1977), hepatitis B subunit (1981), varicella—chickenpox (1981), hepatitis B recombinant (1986), and hepatitis A (1995) (Tulchinsky, 2018).

To elaborate further on his discoveries, through the use of WI-38 cells, he and his team developed "the majority of the 14 vaccines currently recommended for childhood routine immunization and [also] led in the development of other vaccines'" (Tulchinsky, 2018, p. 448). Additionally, as an extension of the work of Baruch and Blumberg and Wolf Szmuness, in 1981, Hilleman created "a vaccine for hepatitis, which is one of the primary causes of liver cancer" (Maugh, 2005, para. 37). In other words, the hepatitis shot was the first vaccine to protect against cancer. Lastly, in 1983, Hilleman's team found vaccines to protect against 14 types of pneumococcal (pneumonia) bacteria, and after the assistance of Robert Austian, a total of 23 pneumococcal types (Tulchinsky, 2018).

Hilleman Receives the National Medal of Science
Preventing many pandemics, saving countless lives, and discovering foundational findings in the sciences, Hilleman clearly understood the function of diseases and how to cultivate immunity in the human body. Unfortunately, Hilleman never won a Nobel Peace Prize or attained the esteem of Salk and Pasteur, but, in 1988, he was credited the National Medal of Science, the nation's highest honor, by President Reagan (Maugh, 2005). As stated by colleagues and close friends, Maurice Hilleman never sought fame or recognition for his research and many vaccine developments (Hilleman Film Team, 2019).

The world is indebted to Hilleman and his many contributions. He is applauded by the science community for his indispensable findings and devotion to defeating a host of foreign invaders, antigens—whether fungal, viral, or parasitic. As mentioned by Hilleman Film Team (2019), "it is likely that Dr. Hilleman's work has saved more lives worldwide than any other scientist in history" ("About Dr. Hilleman").

Chapter 2: What Is a Vaccine?

Vaccines are one the greatest triumphs of modern medicine. They are designed to be a preventative measure against some of the known infectious agents that are pathogenic to humans. Currently there are over 30 vaccines for 26 mainly viral and bacterial pathogens (Ada, 2005). Vaccines are able to induce a lasting immune response against a specific infectious agent so if the body is exposed to the same agent again, the infection is suppressed before the disease becomes symptomatic (Ada, 2005). This ability has substantially reduced the burden of infectious diseases and between the years 1924 and 2010, an estimated 103 million cases of childhood diseases were prevented in the United States (Iwasaki & Omer, 2020). The World Health Organization (WHO) estimates that 2 - 3 million lives are saved each year by current immunization programs, resulting in a significant reduction in global mortality rate in children under the age of 5 (Pollard & Bijker, 2021). To understand how vaccines work, it is important to first review how the body fights infections.

The Immune System
The immune system is a complex network of cells and proteins that defends the body when viruses or bacteria invade the body and start attacking healthy cells. The human immune system can be split into two subsystems, the innate/ resistance system, and the adaptive system (Clem, 2011). The innate system refers to a variety of continuously functioning

protective measures that provide the first line of defense against infectious agents. The innate immune system refers to the anatomical barriers, such as skin and mucous membranes, which inhibit the entry of toxic agents into the body. It also includes physiological barriers, such as body temperature, fever, enzymes, and proteins responsible for preventing the survival of invasive microorganisms within the body. The innate immune response is a generalized reaction to pathogens, meaning they will react in a predictable pattern for all infections. While this is necessary to prevent the innate system from attacking healthy host cells, it prevents the response from improving after being exposed to illnesses. In the case the innate response is unable to suppress the pathogenic agent, it will activate the adaptive immune system.

The adaptive immune system differs from the innate immune system because it has memory. This means the adaptive response has the ability to respond more rapidly and effectively to pathogens after each subsequent exposure. The two main components of the adaptive immune response are the B-cells/antibodies and T-cells. The B-cells and antibodies are part of antibody-mediated immunity, or humoral immunity, and functions against extracellular infectious agents and toxins. The key process in this component is the B-cells' ability to recognize antigens without the assistance of a T-helper cell. An antigen refers to any molecule that the immune system can produce antibodies against. This immune response is stronger when the B-cell activation is coupled with T-helper cell activation as it results in more effective memory. The stimulated B-cells will mature into plasma cells responsible for creating the antibodies specific to a particular antigen. The antibodies will bind to the antigen, neutralizing the pathogen. The remaining plasma cells will become memory cells that will be stored in the lymph nodes, ready to be activated in case the antigen appears again in the future. The second component of the adaptive immune system is the T-cells which function primarily against intracellular pathogens. There are two types of T-cells: T-helper cells and T-cytotoxic cells. As mentioned previously, the T-helper cells assist B-cells in combating extracellular pathogens. The T-cytotoxic or T-killer cell is a type of white blood cell, responsible for killing cancer cells, infected cells, and damaged cells. It is important to note that only the T-cytotoxic cells make up the cellular immunity component of the adaptive immune system. A significant difference in T-cell function compared to B-cells, is that T-cells only recognize antigens after they have been processed and presented by antigen-presenting cells. Once the T-cells are activated by the antigen-presenting cell, they will multiply to fight the current infection and also create memory T-cells for future exposures. Once the infection is eradicated, the adaptive immune system will now have memory B-cells and memory T-cells stored and ready to be activated to defend against this particular pathogen. This long term, effective immune response is the goal of vaccines and immunizations.

Types of Vaccines
Scientists have taken many approaches to developing vaccines. There are many considerations that need to be explored before creating a vaccine. Knowing if the disease is caused by a virus or bacteria, and how the pathogenic agent infects the cells are critical to designing a vaccine. The geographical region or environmental factors can influence the strain of a virus as well as impact the risk of exposure (Centers for Disease Control and Prevention [CDC], 2018). Additionally, the mode of delivery for vaccinations can differ

geographically due to resource constraints. As of today, vaccines can be divided into five different types (Ada, 2005; CDC, 2018; Pollard & Bijker, 2021):

- *Live, attenuated vaccines*
- *Inactivated vaccines*
- *Subunit vaccines (purified protein, recombinant protein, polysaccharides, peptide)*
- *Conjugate vaccines*
- *Toxoids vaccines*

Live, attenuated vaccines
Live, attenuated vaccines are largely considered the most successful type of vaccines for humans (Ada, 2005; CDC, 2018). The major advantage of using live, attenuated vaccines is that they mimic natural infection in the body (Jang & Seong, 2012). As a result, the immune response produced by the body is able to create a long-lasting immunity to the illness.

As the name suggests, live, attenuated vaccines contain a living version of the virus or bacteria that has been weakened to a state where it is unable to cause serious harm to people with healthy immune systems (CDC, 2018). In some cases, vaccines containing the weakened pathogen, will require multiple doses to produce the desired level of immune response from the body (Pollard & Bijker, 2021). Despite the virus or bacteria being in a weakened state, these types of vaccines can not be taken by people with compromised immune systems. Live viruses still have the potential to replicate in an uncontrollable manner if left unchecked by a proper immune response (Pollard & Bijker, 2021). This unique characteristic may cause minor symptoms in the patient to appear after receiving the vaccine. For example, after the measle vaccination around 5% of the children may develop a rash and up to 15% may develop a fever (Pollard & Bijker, 2021).

A variety of approaches have been used to develop this type of vaccine. For example, the measles, mumps, and rubella vaccines are all developed in tissue cultures and animal hosts until the acceptable balance of loss in virulence and retention of immunogenicity in humans is achieved (Ada, 2005). Another approach can be observed in the development of the polio and rotavirus vaccines. In both cases, a naturally occurring attenuated strain of the viruses have been discovered and used in vaccines with great success. Another popular method used by scientists is to weaken viral and bacterial strains using cold-adaptation. This is achieved by selecting mutants that will grow in low temperatures but will struggle to grow in temperatures above 37∘C (Ada, 2005). In other words, these mutant strains will struggle to multiply in the body and can be easily eradicated by the immune response. This is a common practice seen in the development of the influenza vaccines (Ada, 2005; Pollard & Bijker, 2021).

Some of the major advantages of using the cold-adapted live, attenuated vaccines are its ability to preserve genetic stability of the pathogenic agent, capacity for large gene inserts and potential to provide cross-protection (Pollard & Bijker, 2021). These vaccines have been created successfully for several animal viruses including 12 RNA viruses and 2 DNA viruses. One of the major disadvantages of live, attenuated vaccines is found in the trade off between vaccine safety and viral virulence. Generally, as the safety level of the vaccines increases, the ability of the vaccine to replicate in the host decreases due to the increased weakened state of the live viral agent. The loss in efficacy of the vaccine can result in some vaccines requiring multiple doses in order to be effective. The cold-adaptation method has been proven to allow the construction of live, attenuated vaccines, with high safety levels, while simultaneously maintaining the acceptable level of vaccine efficacy and productivity.

With recent advancements in our genome sequencing technology and a push to create vaccines to combat the rising threat of antibiotic resistant illnesses, there have been breakthroughs in the research field on how to incorporate genetic modification techniques in live, attenuated vaccines (Ada, 2005). For example, in the research of influenza virus strains, there has been success in using the reverse genetic technique to create recombinant influenza strains from cloned cDNAs (Pollard & Bijker, 2021). This allows researchers to quickly design strains carrying mutations in multiple different desired positions of interest. The genes from the multiple mutated strains are then inserted and incorporated into a single live, attenuated viral particle. Once the vaccine is administered, the host's body will produce an immune response against all the mutations included in the modified viral genome. This breakthrough effectively allows the administration of vaccines that will provide immunity against multiple different strains of a highly mutable illness.

Genetic modification is also being used as a method to weaken the live pathogenic agent in the vaccine through the deletion or inactivation of one or more genes (Ada, 2005). This approach has resulted in low virulence strains to be created, while maintaining immunogenicity. These methods have only become possible with our recent advancements in genome sequencing and editing techniques. As our understanding of these methods improve, the level of efficacy from live, attenuated vaccines will also continue to increase.

Inactivated vaccines
Inactivated vaccines are created by killing the virus or bacteria in the vaccine. In contrast to live, attenuated vaccines, inactivated vaccines can be administered to immunocompromised individuals with no risk (Pollard & Bijker, 2021). The inactivation of the virus and bacteria often result in varying vaccine efficacy (Ada, 2005). Therefore, inactivated vaccines are given in larger doses and sometimes require multiple doses to be effective (Ada, 2005; CDC, 2018; Pollard & Bijker, 2021). In general, the initial dose "primes" the immune response without producing protective immunity (Centers for Disease Control and Prevention [CDC], 2020). The subsequent doses produce the protective immune response. In contrast to live vaccines, where the immune response activates both humoral and cellular immunity, inactivated vaccines only produce humoral immunity (Ada, 2005; CDC, 2020). This is due little to no cytotoxic T-cell activation by the vaccine. Another disadvantage of inactivated vaccines is the strength of the antibody immunity tends to diminish over time and may require additional booster doses in the future (CDC, 2020).

Subunit Vaccines
Subunit vaccines are a type of inactivated vaccine that presents a fragment of the pathogen to the immune system. In general, subunit vaccines present one or more antigens to the immune system and can be any molecule such as proteins, peptides or polysaccharides. Since subunit vaccines only contain specific antigens, they greatly reduce the likelihood of adverse reactions (CDC, 2008; Clem, 2011).

Unfortunately, this specificity also increases the difficulty of determining which antigens to use in the vaccine (Clem, 2011). Polysaccharide vaccines are a type of subunit vaccines composed of the long sugar molecule chains typically found coating encapsulated bacteria and are easily recognized by the immune system of older individuals (Ada, 2005). The immune response to pure polysaccharide vaccines is B-cell activation without the assistance of T-helper cells (CDC, 2020). A distinct disadvantage of polysaccharide vaccines can be observed in their inability to be recognized by the immune system in young children under the age of two, typically due to the immaturity of their immune systems. Previously we explained booster shots are required to assist vaccines that only stimulate the antibody mediated immunity. In the case of polysaccharide vaccines, repeat doses do not cause a booster response, further decreasing the effectiveness of these types of vaccines.

Vaccine antigens can also be produced through the use of genetic engineering technology. Vaccines that contain genetically modified antigens are known as recombinant vaccines. Recombinant vaccines have been used in inserting gene segments into live, attenuated pathogens which will stimulate the immune system by mimicking a natural infection (Clem, 2011). Genetic modification has also been used to produce desired antigens in modified yeast cells ranging from hepatitis B surface antigens to HPV capsid proteins (CDC, 2020; Nascimento & Leite, 2012). Most recombinant vaccines administered today are recombinant purified proteins of pathogens. Another type of recombinant vaccines are DNA vaccines and consist of non-replicating plasmids (Nascimento & Leite, 2012). The advantages of all recombinant vaccines are their safety and production costs compared to traditional vaccines. However, most recombinant vaccines present weak immunogenicity when given alone. Therefore, these vaccines are often given in conjunction with adjuvants, which are agents that enhance the immune response (Iwasaki & Omer, 2020; Pollard & Bijker, 2021). Adjuvants stimulate the innate immune system through pattern recognition receptors on antigen-presenting cells (Iwasaki & Omer, 2020). As mentioned previously, antigen-presenting cells are required to activate the T-cytotoxic cell component of the adaptive immune system. Together the recombinant vaccine antigens and adjuvants produce the desired long-lasting immune response (Nascimento & Leite, 2012).

Conjugate Vaccines
Conjugate vaccines are another type of inactivated vaccine and are designed to overcome the disadvantages of polysaccharide vaccines (Ada, 2005). Through a process called conjugation, the polysaccharide is chemically combined with a protein molecule (CDC, 2020; Clem, 2011). The protein antigen is easily recognized by the immune system and simultaneously helps immature immune systems recognize the polysaccharide antigen (CDC, 2008). Another advantage of conjugate vaccines lies in their ability to produce both the antibody-mediated immunity and T-cell activation (Ada, 2005). Activation of both components of the adaptive immune response results in long lasting immunity and has been successful in saving the lives of many young children (Ada, 2005).

Toxoid Vaccines
Toxoid vaccines is another type of inactivated vaccine that are used to prevent diseases caused by toxins produced by

bacteria (CDC, 2008). The toxins directly promote infection by damaging host cells and interfering with the immune system. These vaccines are produced by weakening or inactivating the toxins with formalin, to prevent the illness from becoming symptomatic (CDC, 2008; Clem, 2011). When toxoid vaccines are administered, the immune system is stimulated to fight the bacterial toxins (Clem, 2011). In general, toxoid vaccines only contain the toxoid, weakened disease causing toxin, instead of the bacteria itself. This allows toxoid vaccines to be extremely safe and effective and administered as part of routine childhood vaccinations against diseases such as the diphtheria, tetanus and whooping cough (pertussis). Similar to all the other types of inactivated vaccines, toxoid vaccines also require several doses in order to be effective.

Vaccines Mechanism of Action

There are many different vaccines currently being administered around the world and each of them may result in varying levels of protection against specific diseases. However, the one common fact of all vaccines is they are responsible for creating active immunity. Unlike passive immunity, which is temporary, active immunity can last multiple years to provide protection for a lifetime. The introduction of a novel antigen in the body, whether it is in the form of a live but weakened version of the infectious agent, a bacterial toxin, or an inactivated fragment of the pathogen, all cause the immune system to react in the same way. The first component of the adaptive immune system, which is the production of B-cells, will be activated (CDC, 2020). As mentioned earlier stimulated B-cells will produce antibodies to bind and inactivate the antigens (Clem, 2011). Many factors will influence the level of immune response including the dosage, method of administration, and if there was an adjuvant included (CDC, 2020). Inactivated and subunit vaccines when administered without adjuvants require multiple doses to fully activate the antibody-mediated immunity (Ada, 2005; CDC, 2018; Pollard & Bijker, 2021). Inactivated vaccines produce a relatively weak immunity and require booster doses in the future to maintain the desired level of memory B-lymphocytes levels in the body (CDC, 2020). Subunit vaccines, such as polysaccharides vaccines, can only produce antibody-mediated immunity that steadily declines over time and is unable to be boosted with additional doses. With the inclusion of adjuvants in subunit vaccines, the innate immune response is activated and produces antigen presenting cells (Iwasaki & Omer, 2020). These cells play a critical role in activating the T-cytotoxic cells of the adaptive immune response ((Iwasaki & Omer, 2020; Pollard & Bijker, 2021). This results in both components of the adaptive immune response to be activated and fosters the long-term immunity desired from vaccines (Nascimento & Leite, 2012). Recombinant vaccines and live, attenuated vaccines are able to activate the cellular immunity component of the adaptive immune response without the need of adjuvants. These types of vaccines activate the sufficient level of memory T-lymphocytes and B-lymphocytes that produce the long lasting immunity responsible for saving millions of lives every year.

It is important to understand that the body's immune response takes several days to activate and fight off a novel infection. Furthermore, it may take weeks before memory T-lymphocytes and B-lymphocytes are produced (CDC, 2018). In the case of vaccines that require booster shots or multiple doses, the desired level of immunity may take months after the initial dose to be achieved. The goal of vaccines is to safely produce the memory B-lymphocytes and T-lymphocytes in the body with little to no risk to the host. Therefore on subsequent infection by the illness, the body will be equipped with the tools to eradicate the disease efficiently.

Chapter 3: Testing and Trials

What is a Clinical Trial?
A clinical trial is a research study where the effectiveness of
a treatment for a disease or disorder is tested using human
volunteers as test subjects (U.S. Food & Drug Administration,
2014). The clinical trials will test either a new treatment or
compare a new discovery to similar treatments used in the
past. Different ways a treatment can be used will be tested as
well, so that there could potentially be different uses of the
procedure depending on people's conditions, thus measuring
the participants' reactions when determining the safety
of the treatment. This is a critical step to take in a medical
intervention as the integration of the treatment with humans
has to be thoroughly assessed before mass production.
This reduces the risk of any side effects occurring in a large
number of people. When correctly carried out, clinical trials
are the safest and the most efficient way to find answers
to particular questions regarding health and methods of
improving it.

Types of Clinical Trials
Depending on what researchers wish to test, as well as on
how the test is designed, there are several types of clinical
trials (U.S. National Library of Medicine, 2019). Firstly,
clinical trials can either be therapeutic or non-therapeutic.
A therapeutic trial is where the treatment being tested
has already been designed and is in the experimental

stage. Therefore, there is hope from researchers that the experimental treatment will benefit the research participants in some way. A non-therapeutic trial's sole purpose is for researchers to obtain further information on a treatment in order to commence the design and develop the treatment. Due to this, a non-therapeutic trial is not expected to be of any benefit to the test subjects involved in the study.

Next, a clinical trial can be classified into four types: treatment trials, prevention trials, observational trials, and diagnostic trials:

Treatment trial
A clinical trial with a goal to test treatments that have not yet been approved as they are still in the experimental stage. These treatments can include either medication aimed to cure the condition being treated, or medication intended to manage any symptoms that accompany the condition being treated.

Prevention trial
This trial aims to test several methods to prevent certain diseases or disorders, as well as their symptoms or recurrences.

Observational trial
The purpose is to analyze the medical conditions for which a medical intervention is being planned. Researchers will ask participants who are diagnosed with the condition being studied several questions regarding their individual experiences with their health issue. Depending on the objective of the study, test subjects will be asked to provide other information such as a blood sample or urine sample.

Diagnostic trial
This trial strives to find more efficient ways to detect a disease or disorder, so that the treatment of the medical condition is more prompt and thorough.

How do Clinical Trials Work?

Clinical trials follow a protocol, a plan according to which it must be thoroughly conducted. When researchers carry out clinical trials, they must make it very clear to participants, and ultimately the public, what the study requires and consists of. When selecting research participants, those conducting the clinical trials must make it clear what physical or medical state is recommended for an individual to be in when carrying out the trial. This is to determine what patient group to avoid or to target depending on what medical treatment is being tested. Once test subjects have been selected for the clinical trial, researchers must communicate the design and reasoning behind the treatments, and emphasize other additional information such as the dosages they plan to administer, what schedule they will follow when administering the dosages, and for how long the clinical trial is intended to last. This ensures that all research participants are fully aware of what they are agreeing to, while holding researchers accountable throughout the duration of the clinical trial.

Phases in a Clinical Trial

Clinical trials need to be carried out in phases, for the sake of cost efficiency as well as the safety of the individuals participating in the study. For each stage, data is collected and thoroughly reviewed to determine if the aimed effect of the treatment has been acquired while ensuring the well-being of the research participants is being prioritized. Clinical trials for vaccines typically take approximately six to twelve months or longer due to how much clinical trials cost, however, desired results can be achieved earlier on (Griffin, 2020, p. 1).

Before a clinical trial for a vaccine, it must go through a preclinical phase. This means that the vaccine is tested on animals who share similar DNA as humans, such as cattle or rats. Animal testing helps to determine if there are any toxicities induced by the vaccine that would prevent it from being distributed to humans. Systemic reactions including immune reactions to the vaccine as well as reactions at the injection site will be assessed. Once enough data is collected, researchers and ethics committees must approve of the safety and the efficacy of the vaccine in the animal studies, then the vaccine may begin its clinical trial with humans as the test subjects in the study.

A clinical trial that is designed for a vaccine is split into four phases:

Phase 1
This phase of a vaccine clinical trial usually consists of a quite small population with a smaller range of diversity as the level of safety that was confirmed in the preclinical stage needs to be confirmed once more before continuing the study. This trial is carried out in a laboratory setting and researchers analyze the interaction between blood samples of research participants and the vaccine. This way, doses can be altered in a safe manner according to how the immune system will react to the vaccine as being seen in the blood samples.

Phase 2
Similarly to phase 1, this phase still has a primary focus on

the safety of the research participants. The interaction of the vaccine in given blood samples will still be assessed but with a larger and more diverse population. This will give a better understanding of how the vaccine will interact with different medical conditions involved, and also give insight as to how different age ranges can play a role in how the body reacts to certain doses of a vaccine being administered. At this stage, researchers are still unable to confirm the efficacy of the vaccine being tested or if the goals of the research have been achieved. Therefore, it is necessary to have additional phases to follow up in a clinical trial for a vaccine.

Phase 3
This phase requires a much larger group of participants because this is the stage where the vaccine will be approved for mass production and use, or if there needs to be further adjustment before approval. In this phase, researchers see if there is any significant change in the conditions of research participants, such as lower rates of being infected by the disease the vaccine was designed to treat.

Phase 4
The last phase of a clinical trial for a vaccine, this is the stage where the vaccine is being used by a vast population, and data regarding its effect on the health of the public continues to be recorded and reviewed.

The Approval Process
The approval process for a vaccine in development is just as lengthy as that of the clinical trials. Vaccines are a distinctive form of treatment as they are considered to be both a drug and a biological product (Walter & Moody, 2021, p. 1). A drug is a substance that is used to diagnose, cure, mitigate,

treat and prevent diseases. The primary difference between a drug and a biological product is that drugs are made from and synthesized with chemical structures, while biological products are derived from living organisms. Biological products are "complex mixtures composed of sugars, proteins, nucleic acids, or complex combinations of these substances, or they may be living entities such as cells and tissues" (Walter & Moody, 2021, p. 1). Therefore, drugs are only meant to be prescribed and administered to individuals who have been diagnosed with medical illnesses, while biological products such as vaccines can be given to any individual. Their safety in comparison to drugs, whether prescribed or over the counter, is why adults and children alike are able to be given doses of various vaccines as a preventative measure. Given their universal and essential use, heavy regulations are required during the development, approval, and distribution stages of the vaccine in order to guarantee public safety.

During the last stages of vaccine clinical trials, the investigational vaccine is being evaluated for consistency across different manufacturing sites, safety and immunogenicity, and the "ability of an antigen to provoke an immune response" (Walter & Moody, 2021, p. 3). These assessments will allow the investigational vaccine to be tested with other vaccines that have already been approved in order to determine whether they can be coadministered. Once these final evaluations have been completed, the vaccine approval process can begin.

To ensure complete safety of the general population, the vaccines are meticulously monitored and adjusted until they can be approved. Different countries have their own regulations when it comes to their approval process for vaccines. In this chapter, the approval processes in the United States of America and Canada will be discussed.

Vaccine Approval in the United States of America
In the United States of America, vaccine sponsors, those who are funding the production of the vaccines, can file a Biologics License Application (BLA) with the Food and Drug Administration (FDA). By filing this application, sponsors are requesting permission to advance the biological product they developed to interstate commerce. Vaccine sponsors must include information in their Biologics License Application such as "applicant information, product and manufacturing information, preclinical and clinical study data, and proposed product labelling information" (Walter & Moody, 2021, p. 3). The purpose of the product label is to explain to healthcare providers the objectives of the vaccine, its possible benefits and risks, as well as instructions on how to store the vaccine and how the vaccine is meant to be administered. The Food and Drug Administration will then visit the vaccine manufacturing plants in order to conduct a thorough inspection of the manufacturing process for the investigational vaccine. This amount of detailed information regarding the investigational vaccine will allow the Food and Drug Administration team to conduct a proper assessment of the risks and benefits of the potential distribution of this vaccine.

Upon reviewing the license application, the FDA and the vaccine sponsor will present the findings from the evaluations to the Vaccines and Related Biological Products Advisory Committee (VRBPAC) of the Food and Drugs Administration. This committee is a "non-FDA expert committee" that "provides advice regarding the safety and efficacy of the vaccine for the proposed indication and assists the FDA with its determination for approval of the vaccine" (Walter & Moody, 2021, p. 3).

Once the Food and Drug Administration approves of and grants a license to the investigational vaccine, the Advisory Committee on Immunization Practices (ACIP) of the Centers for Disease Control and Prevention (CDC) advises sponsors on how the vaccine should be used when being administered to civilians of the United States of America. The committee takes many factors into consideration such as how effective the vaccine is, how safe it is, and how it will proceed to interact with the immune system. Other important factors that are taken into consideration are how severe the disease(s) being treated by the vaccine is(are) and how many people could potentially contract the disease(s) if there was no vaccine distribution.

After the FDA has approved the vaccine and has allowed public distribution, the safety of the vaccine and how it interacts with people still continues to be monitored. This is to ensure that the previously investigated vaccine continues to be safe and thoroughly effective.

Vaccine Approval in Canada
In Canada, the health care system and the government alike play a significant role in the development, regulation, and the process of authorizing a vaccine under investigation. Five main groups are: Health Canada, the Public Health Agency of Canada (PHAC) reported to by the National Advisory Committee on Immunization, provincial and territorial health authorities, and health care providers (Government of Canada, 2011).

Health Canada regulates vaccine production by using clinical evidence to conclude the quality and safety of a vaccine undergoing clinical trials. Therefore, this organization will only authorize high quality vaccines that are effective and safe. Upon authorizing vaccines for sale, the vaccines being sold will be closely supervised to ensure their consistent quality and effectiveness.

The Public Health Agency of Canada is responsible for providing the public with information regarding the immunization process and the types of vaccines that are being administered. The Agency uses the Canadian Adverse Events Following Immunization Surveillance System (CAEFISS) to keep track of the safety of the vaccines, vaccine failures following immunization, and certain infectious diseases that are able to be averted due to vaccination (Government of Canada).

The National Advisory Committee on Immunization reports to the Public Health Agency of Canada, revising submitted evidence of the efficacy and the lack of side effects in approved vaccines in order to make recommendations to the Agency regarding the proper use of approved vaccines (Government of Canada).

Health authorities in the Canadian provinces and territories determine what immunization schedule their region should follow, while also ensuring health care providers accurately report what occurs in the population after getting vaccinated. They place an emphasis on the cruciality of reporting all unfavorable events that occur following immunization (Government of Canada).

Finally, health care providers are the people who administer vaccines to their patients while keeping them informed of important details regarding the vaccine. They are also responsible for reporting to their local public health unit if any adverse events occur after a patient has been vaccinated (Government of Canada).

The approval process for a vaccine in Canada is similar to that in the United States. First, if researchers and manufacturers wish to perform a clinical trial on an investigational vaccine, they must submit a Clinical Trial Application to Health Canada's Biologic and Radiopharmaceutical Drug Directorate. This is to evaluate the quality of the products being tested and ensure that no harm will come to clinical trial subjects within the duration of the study.

Once enough proof of safety has been obtained, manufacturers are able to file a New Drug Submission where they can display this evidence along with how the vaccine will be manufactured, where the manufacturing facility is, and how the manufacturers intend to monitor the quality of the vaccine (Government of Canada). Upon obtaining the submission, Health Canada will determine how effective the vaccine is while it is being developed. The vaccine must prove that it will be an effective enough treatment with the benefits overlaying any safety concerns that may hinder the approval of the investigational vaccine. Health Canada will proceed to ask manufacturers to provide prototypes of the vaccine under investigation to confirm that vaccines of high quality will consistently be produced.

Before the investigational vaccine is officially authorized for sale, Health Canada's Biological and Radiopharmaceutical

Drugs Directorate will review the data shown in the New Drug Submission (Government of Canada). When it is confirmed that there are no great safety concerns regarding the investigational vaccine, Health Canada will provide a Notice of Compliance (NOC) and a Drug Identification Number (DIN) (Government of Canada). This confirms that the vaccine that underwent clinical trials has been authorized to be sold in the country.

All vaccines that have been authorized in Canada enter a lot released program where the quality of the vaccine continues to be monitored to test for consistency (Government of Canada). Upon meeting all of the requirements, Health Canada's Biological and Radiopharmaceutical Drug Directorate will issue a formal release letter for the vaccine lot to be officially approved for sale in Canada (Government of Canada).

The following two chapters will discuss vaccines in a more relevant manner in regards to the current coronavirus global pandemic: what is COVID-19, what sorts of vaccines are needed to effectively treat the disease, and how are they being used?

Chapter 4: What Is COVID-19?

On January 30 2020, the World Health Organization (WHO) declared COVID-19 to be a Public Health Emergency of International Concern (PHEIC), and only a month and a half later on March 11 2020, they declared it a global pandemic. Governments around the world quickly responded by implementing lockdowns which included closing public spaces, stay-at-home orders, travel restrictions, and social distancing measures in hopes of curbing the spread of the virus. As of May 15, 2021 – over a year into the pandemic – there have been approximately 161.5 million confirmed COVID-19 cases and 3.4 million confirmed COVID-19 deaths reported to WHO (2021). The lockdowns have eased in some countries while others continue to hold alternating periods of loosened and heightened restrictions as cases slow and surge. The COVID-19 pandemic is a global event that has had a drastic impact on all of our lives and brought with it immense change to the world around us. But what exactly is COVID-19? This chapter will aim to give an overview of COVID-19 and explain the mechanisms by which it infects and spreads.

Background
Coronaviruses are a group of viruses found in humans and other animals that are known to cause respiratory, gastrointestinal, and neurological disease (Wiersinga et al., 2020). COVID-19, which is short for coronavirus disease 2019, is the disease that is caused by the SARS-CoV-2 virus.

Short for severe acute respiratory syndrome coronavirus 2, SARS-CoV-2 was first detected in Wuhan, Hubei in December of 2019 and was eventually named as such due to its shared homology with the coronavirus responsible for the SARS epidemic in 2003, SARS-CoV (Dos Santos 2020). SARS-CoV-2 and SARS-CoV along with another coronavirus, Middle East respiratory syndrome CoV (MERS-CoV) which had an epidemic outbreak in 2012, are the three zoonotic CoV viruses detected in humans to date (Catanzaro et al., 2020). This means that these viruses were not present in the human population until a spillover event from a reservoir host animal occurred (Public Health Ontario, 2020). Although the definite animal source for SARS-CoV-2 is still unconfirmed, research thus far has heavily suggested that the virus originated from horseshoe bats due to a 96% genetic proximity between SARS-CoV-2 and RaTG13, a bat sarbecovirus (Boni et al., 2020). Pangolins have also been implicated as a potential intermediate host of the virus due to similarity of key binding residues between the pangolin coronavirus strain and SARS-CoV-2 – something that is not seen between the RaTG13 and SARS-CoV-2 (Boni et al., 2020; Mackenzie and Smith, 2020). Thus, it is probable that the origin of SARS-CoV-2 is more complex than initially thought and may have included a recombination event between the pangolin CoV and RaTG13 (Mackenzie and Smith, 2020; Wong et al., 2020).

Infection

To understand how SARS-CoV-2 infects and attacks the body, one must first understand its structure. As with other coronaviruses, SARS-CoV-2 contains crown-like spike proteins on its envelope, hence the name "corona" (Ouassou et al., 2020). It is 65-125 nm in diameter and contains a positive-sense single-stranded RNA virus as nucleic material

(Ouassou et al., 2020). Although spherical in shape, a concave surface with a ridge on one side increases binding area and affinity (Chowdhury et al., 2020). Receptor-binding domains (RBD) in the spike proteins on the virus's surface recognize angiotensin-converting enzyme 2 (ACE2) in host cells as their receptor (Shang et al., 2020). In humans, once the virus is inhaled, it uses these spike proteins to bind to the ACE2 of epithelial cells in the nasal cavity and endocytosis of the virus occurs (Mason, 2020; Oliveira et al., 2020). The virus then propagates by releasing its viral RNA and hijacking the host cell machinery to produce progeny virions which then transfer viral RNA to new host cells (Faisst, 1999; Oliveira et al., 2020). At this stage, the virus can be detected through a test and may be spread to other individuals, although infected individuals will still be asymptomatic (Mason, 2020).

The virus makes its way down the respiratory tract at which point individuals will experience the clinical manifestation of the virus, COVID-19. A stronger immune system response is activated and 80% of individuals will have infection limited to upper and conducting airways, only experiencing mild symptoms similar to the common cold such as fever, dry coughing, sore throat, fatigue, aches, diarrhea, and shortness of breath (Mason, 2020; Wiersinga et al., 2020). However, 20% of infected individuals will be more vulnerable to the virus and will experience symptoms of higher severity, such as difficulty breathing, chest pain, and loss of speech or movement (Esakandari et al., 2020). These individuals will experience the development of disease, severe pneumonia, and even death in some cases (Catanzaro et al., 2020). Individuals in this higher risk, vulnerable category may include older aged adults, males, obese individuals, and those with pre-existing lung disease, heart conditions, diabetes mellitus, or cancer (Kommoss et al., 2020).

The virus may move to the lungs, where lung alveoli which are generously covered in ACE2 receptors are brutally attacked (Wadman et al., 2020). Not only does this disrupt healthy oxygen flow through the body, but the immune response to these attacks can become excessive and dysregulated (Wadman et al., 2020). An increase in pro-inflammatory cytokines and chemokines (also known as a "cytokine storm") can contribute to lung damage and organ failure as immune cells mistakenly attack healthy tissue (Oliveria et al., 2020; Catanzaro et al., 2020). Chemokines also provoke more immune cells to pick out and destroy virus-infected cells, causing alveoli to become filled with pus composed of dead cells, mucus, and fluid, potentially leading to pneumonia and acute respiratory distress syndrome (ARDS) (Wadman et al., 2020). This immune system activation is followed by an immune system suppression, where the risk of bacterial infection is increased (Gavriatopoulo et al,. 2020). This is caused by lymphopenia, where lymphocytes - a type of white blood cell and key player in immune defense - are decreased in the blood (Gavriatopoulo et al., 2020).

As well, it is important to note that although COVID-19 is primarily a respiratory illness, other organs in the body are not free from impact. The virus can bind to the ACE2 receptors of different cell types in areas besides the lungs such as the heart, brain, kidneys, liver, gastrointestinal tract, and pharynx and cause damage (Jain, 2020). The hyperinflammation resulting from the body's immune response and cytokine storm can also contribute to organ damage in these areas (Gavriatopoulo et al., 2020). Indeed, there have been cases of COVID-19 induced myocarditis (inflammation of the heart muscle which can reduce pumping ability, cause abnormal rhythms, and weaken the heart) confirming the threat that COVID-19 poses for cardiac injury (Gavriatopoulo et al., 2020; Myocarditis Foundation, n.d.). Correlations have also been found between COVID-19 and nervous system injury. Some infected patients have reported symptoms including dizziness, headaches, loss of taste, impaired consciousness and vision, nerve pain, strokes, and seizures (Gavriatopoulo et al., 2020). The virus may also damage nerve endings in the nose and result in the loss of a sense of smell, something that has been reported by many COVID-19 patients (Wadman et al., 2020).

It was previously mentioned that older adults are at a higher risk of developing severe symptoms and disease. Indeed, Mueller et al. (2020) reported age to be the most significant risk factor of COVID-19 induced death, but why is this? Multiple hypotheses exist. Aging is associated with declines in many areas of health. An area of particular importance due to the current COVID-19 pandemic is immunity. As individuals age, they face immune system efficacy deterioration. Epithelial barriers in the skin, lungs, and digestive track erode and allow for easier pathogen access, pathogen recognition and antibody quality decreases, memory lymphocytes become anergic, the ability of T and B cells to fend off infections is weakened, chronic inflammation damages organs in the body, and vaccine efficacy is reduced (Whaley et al., 2019; Schenkelberg, 2021; Mueller et al., 2020). Such changes are encompassed by the term immunosenescence. Immunosenescence is not only attributed to normal, primary aging, but can be exacerbated by poor cumulative lifestyle choices and environmental factors (Whaley et al., 2019). It is associated with increased vulnerability to infection and can thus explain why older adults are at a higher risk for severe COVID-19 manifestations (Solana and Pawelec, 2004).

Additionally, older adults infected with COVID-19 may be more likely to undergo the deleterious cytokine storm due to an age-related increase in NLRP3, a protein component of inflammasome, which induces inflammation in response to pathogens (Mueller et al., 2020; Davis et al., 2014). Indeed, data has shown the disproportionate effect of COVID-19 on older adults. According to the CDC, 8 out of 10 COVID-19 deaths have been in individuals aged 65 and older. As well, the CDC has reported that compared to 18-29 year olds, those aged 65-74 are 90 times more likely to die from COVID-19. For individuals above the age of 85, these mortality likelihoods jump to 630 times higher. While only 0.3% of infected 40 year olds will die from COVID-19, 13.4% of infected 80 year olds will die from COVID-19 (Lam et al., 2020). Just as older adults, obese individuals and diabetics also have increased activity of NLRP3 and experience hyperactivity of inflammasome, respectively, thus also predisposing these individuals to cytokine storms which increase the risk of mortality (Mueller et al., 2020).

Variants
Since the COVID-19 pandemic began, concerns regarding variants of SARS-CoV-2 have garnered significant attention from the media and the scientific community. But what exactly is a variant, how does it arise, and why is it worrying? As mentioned previously, SARS-CoV-2 is an RNA virus. RNA viruses are more prone to mutation than DNA viruses are (Lauring and Hodcroft, 2021). This is because RNA synthesis does not have the same proofreading functions and repair mechanisms that are seen in DNA synthesis, leading to

random changes in the genomic sequence of the virus during replication that go unfixed (Domingo, 1997). Mutations that give the virus a competitive advantage will be naturally selected for and increase in frequency (Lauring and Hodcroft, 2021). Specifically, mutations that result in greater viral replication, higher transmission, or better ability to escape the immune response will increase in frequency (Lauring and Hodcroft, 2021). In contrast, mutations that lead to decreased fitness of the virus will decrease in frequency as they are selected against (Lauring and Hodcroft, 2021). However, it is important to note that not all mutations will result in an altered fitness. For example, 4000 mutations of the SARS-CoV-2 spike protein have already been identified by researchers, but most do not change the fitness of the virus (Hossain et al., 2021). Additionally, genetic drift - a driver of evolution caused by chance events - is another factor that can contribute to a change in frequency of a mutation (Lauring and Hodcroft, 2021).

Variants, then, are simply versions of the virus that have genomes which differ in sequence as a result of mutations (Lauring and Hodcroft, 2021). Not all variants are strains, however. Even though a variant may have a different genotype from the wild-type SARS-CoV-2, it only becomes classified as a new strain when it displays a different phenotype - an observable characteristic or behaviour (Lauring and Hodcroft, 2021). An example of this would be a variant demonstrating higher transmissibility. Despite this distinction, the terms variant and strain are often used interchangeably. In December of 2020, reported cases of COVID-19 rose unexpectedly due to new SARS-CoV-2 variants, 501Y.V1 (B.1.1.7) and 501Y.V2 (B.1.351), emerging in the United Kingdom and South Africa, respectively (Fontanet et al., 2021). Both of these variants had D614G and N501Y mutations in the receptor-binding domain of the spike protein, allowing them to interact more efficiently with the ACE2 receptor and consequently giving them increased transmission ability (Mascola et al., 2021; Fontanet et al., 2021). The United Kingdom 501Y.V1 or B.1.1.7 variant was also found to have two other mutations in its spike protein, E484K and K417N, which allow for the variant to potentially escape host immune system antibodies (Fontanet et al., 2021). Research has suggested that this strain is 30-80% more effectively transmitted and offers a 30% increased risk of death compared to the wild-type SARS-CoV-2 strain (Mascola et al., 2021). It also has a reproduction number (R) of 1.45, whereas the wild-type SARS-CoV-2 only has an R value of 0.92 (Hossain et al., 2021). Indeed, despite first being identified in only the United Kingdom, by April 25, 2021, the 501Y.V1/B.1.1.7 had already been transmitted to over 50 countries (Hossain et al., 2021). At the same time, the South Africa 501Y.V2/B.1.351 variant had spread to over twenty (Hossain et al., 2021).

Variants also have different classifications; a variant may be defined as a variant of interest (VOI), a variant of concern (VOC), or a variant of high consequence (VOHC). According to the CDC, VOIs are variants with genetic markers that are associated with increased fitness, transmissibility, disease severity, or ability to escape diagnosis, immunity, or treatment. They are the cause of an unexpected increase in cases or the source of a cluster of cases, but they are not prevalent in the United States and in other countries. VOCs are variants which have shown evidence of these characteristics and will require more drastic public health action. This may involve efforts to control and contain the spread of the variant, increased diagnostic efforts, or adjustments to vaccines and treatments in order to combat the VOC. In addition to the B.1.1.7 and B.1.351 variants, the CDC has also currently classified variants B.1.427, B.1.429, and P.1 as VOCs. VOHCs have been defined by the CDC as variants which have "clear evidence that prevention measures or medical countermeasures (MCMs) have significantly reduced effectiveness relative to previously circulating variants". VOHCs may lead to severe disease and increase risk of hospitalization and treatments against the VOHC will have greatly reduced efficacy. Currently, no SARS-CoV-2 variants have been classified as VOHCs.

The longer an outbreak lasts, the more individuals are infected, and the more opportunities the virus has to spread and mutate, creating more variants. These variants then undergo natural selection, where stronger strains increase in frequency and spread even more, infecting more individuals and creating the potential for an epidemic rebound (Fontanet et al., 2021). This highlights the importance of controlling the spread of a virus as early as possible by adhering to proper public safety guidelines.

Long-Term Effects
Despite recovery, many COVID-19 survivors remain afflicted with persisting symptoms such as fatigue, muscle weakness, sleep problems, depression, or anxiety (Huang et al., 2021). Ninety-five days after first showing symptoms of COVID-19, Paul Garner, a professor of epidemiology at the Liverpool School of Tropical Medicine, shared that he was still experiencing extreme fatigue, had trouble getting out of bed, ringing in his ears, brain fog, and dramatic mood swings (Yelin et al., 2020). He was not alone in his

struggles, in one study by Carfi et al. (2020), 143 COVID-19 survivors were surveyed for any persisting symptoms they may have been experiencing, and 87.4% reported at least one persisting symptom - the most common ones including fatigue, shortness of breath, joint pain, chest pain, cough, and loss of smell. A meta-analysis by Lopez-Leon et al. (2021) found similar results. The meta-analysis examined 15 studies relating to long-term COVID-19 effects and found 80% of recovered patients were still experiencing at least one persistent symptom - with the most common ones including fatigue (58%), headache (44%), attention disorder (27%), hair loss (25%), and shortness of breath (24%). Lastly, 34% of patients also had abnormal chest x-rays/CTs. The long-term effects of COVID-19 will require continual research and monitoring in order to help patients reestablish their pre-COVID health.

Transmission

Transmission of SARS-CoV-2 mainly occurs after an infected individual breathes, sneezes, coughs, shouts, or talks and produces microscopic respiratory droplets (aerosols) which are inhaled by another individual or come into contact with their nasal, oral, or eye mucous membranes (Government of Canada, 2021). However, these droplets are generally restricted to a radius of six feet around an infected individual, hence the six foot social distancing guideline suggested by the Centers for Disease Control and Prevention (CDC) (Lofti et al,. 2020; Centers for Disease Control and Prevention, 2021). Physical contact with contaminated surfaces can also indirectly cause transmission, although the airborne route is dominant (Lofti et al., 2020). As well, the virus may remain in the air for up to three hours (Lofti et al., 2020). For these reasons, the CDC and WHO have recommended wearing face masks that cover the nose and mouth and many governments have made the usage of these masks in public spaces a legal requirement (World Health Organization, 2021; Centers for Disease Control and Prevention, 2021). However, masks alone are not considered enough to protect oneself from the virus. SARS-CoV-2 has a higher binding efficacy than SARS-CoV, thus making it more transmissible and explaining the difference in magnitude of the two outbreaks (Gavriatopoulo et al., 2020). COVID-19 has also been found to spread more efficiently than influenza (Centers for Disease Control and Prevention, 2021). Therefore, the CDC and WHO have also recommended washing hands regularly, using sanitizer, avoiding public spaces, limiting contact with others, and keeping rooms well ventilated for extra protection against the high contagiousness of SARS-CoV-2 (World Health Organization, 2021; Centers for Disease Control and Prevention, 2021).

Treatment
Being a respiratory illness, many of the treatments targeted at alleviating the manifestations of COVID-19 have been aimed at maintaining and improving lung function. Seventy-five percent of infected patients who are hospitalized are administered supplemental oxygen therapy (Wiersinga et al., 2020). Severe cases may require the use of mechanical ventilation (Wiersinga et al., 2020). Many drugs have also been explored as treatment options for COVID-19. Among them, Remdesivir has shown to be the most promising and is currently the only antiviral drug approved by the Food and Drug Administration (FDA) for the treatment of COVID-19 (Jean et al., 2020; National Institutes of Health, 2021). Remdesivir targets viral RNA-dependent RNA polymerase to terminate the viral RNA transcription and stop propagation of the virus (Jean et al., 2020). Another drug, Dexamethasone,

is a corticosteroid that has been used and shown promise for improving the survival of infected patients who have progressed to the point of requiring mechanical ventilation, since Remdesivir has not shown to benefit patients at this advanced stage as it does to those who only require supplemental oxygen (National Institutes of Health, 2021). Dexamethasone works to suppress the hyperinflammatory immune response, thus it is not useful for patients only in the mild or moderate stages of COVID-19 (National Institutes of Health, 2021). Indeed, researchers have been wary of attempts to reduce the cytokine storm and inflammation as it may end up allowing for more viral replication as the necessary immune response needed by the body to fight off infection is diminished by intervention (Wadman et al., 2020).

For infected patients who are not hospitalized but are in a high risk category, the use of anti-SARS-CoV-2 monoclonal antibodies has been recommended (National Institutes of Health, 2021). Combinations of bamlanivimab and etesevimad, or casirivimab and imdevimad, although unapproved, have been given Emergency Use Authorization for COVID-19 by the FDA (National Institutes of Health, 2021; Food and Drug Administration, 2021). These monoclonal antibodies are lab-manufactured, but act similarly to our natural antibodies, working to help the immune system recognize and respond to the virus (Food and Drug Administration, 2021). For infected patients who are not hospitalized nor in a high risk category, simple supportive care and symptomatic management has been recommended (National Institutes of Health, 2021). This may include taking ibuprofen or acetaminophen, staying hydrated, and resting in order to support the body's natural defenses (Centers for Disease Control and Prevention, 2021). Geroprotectors have also been explored as a way to combat the deterioration of the immune system in aging individuals and thus defend against infections such as COVID-19. However, given the high mortality rates despite the ongoing use of oxygen and drug therapies, it is clear that the solution to this pandemic lies within vaccines. The next chapter will dive into the current COVID-19 vaccines being administered and explain how they work as well as the differences between each.

Chapter 5: The COVID-19 Vaccines Administered

With the onset of the COVID-19 pandemic, there ensued a race within the scientific community to develop a vaccine and control the spread of SARS-CoV-2. Since this race began, over 300 vaccine projects have been developed and many clinical evaluations and trials have commenced. Vaccination will provide individuals with protection against the virus by enabling them to build immunity towards it. On a larger scale, once enough people are vaccinated, the global population will ideally be able to reach herd immunity, where enough individuals are immune to COVID-19 to control its spread by reducing transmission from individual to individual, creating indirect protection even for those who are not immune. The percentage of the population needing to be immune to reach herd immunity varies with each disease. However, for COVID-19, experts estimate that we will need at least 70% of the population to be immune, assuming new, more infectious variants of SARS-CoV-2 do not arise (D'Souza and Dowdy, 2021). Thanks to the combined efforts of countless researchers, there are now a few COVID-19 vaccines that have completed their clinical phases and have been approved for emergency use, bringing us closer to this goal of ending the pandemic and returning to our normal lives. The Food and Drug Administration (FDA) has so far authorized the Pfizer-BioNTech, Moderna, and Janssen (commonly referred to as the Johnson & Johnson vaccine) vaccines for emergency use. Canada has also approved these three, as well as the Oxford-

AstraZeneca/COVISHIELD vaccine. This chapter will give an overview of these vaccines as well as Sinovac's CoronaVac vaccine, which has been approved for use in China (and other countries) and the Novavax vaccine and explore the differences between them.

The Different Vaccines

Pfizer and Moderna
The Pfizer-BioNTech (Tozinameran or BNT162b2) and Moderna (mRNA-1273) vaccines are anti-SARS-CoV-2 messenger ribonucleic acid (mRNA) vaccines. The development of the Pfizer-BioNTech vaccine was started in January of 2020 by BioNTech, a German based biotechnology and immunotherapy company (Corum and Zimmer, 2021). Pfizer, an American biotechnology and pharmaceutical company, later agreed to collaborate on the vaccine in March of 2020. The vaccine was sent to the FDA for Emergency Use Authorization on November 20th, 2020 and was granted it on December 11th, 2020. In Canada, the vaccine was authorized just a few days earlier on December 9th, 2020. Moderna, Inc., another American biotechnology and pharmaceutical company focused on pioneering and developing mRNA therapeutics, similarly began their work on a COVID-19 vaccine in January of 2020. In March of 2020, they became the first developers to begin human trials for a COVID-19 vaccine. The vaccine was sent to the FDA for Emergency Use Authorization on November 30th, 2020 and was granted it on December 18th, 2020. Canada approved the vaccine shortly after, on December 23rd, 2020.

These were the first mRNA-based vaccines to be authorized for use on the general healthy population (Cao and Gao,

2021). Rather than using live viruses, mRNA vaccines simply contain genetic information that provides our cells with instructions on how to make a protein that will trigger an immune response (Government of Canada, 2021). Using liposomes (lipid microvesicles), the Pfizer and Moderna vaccines deliver synthetic mRNA to our cells in order to temporarily induce the cell to produce SARS-CoV-2 spike proteins coded by the mRNA (Forni and Mantovani, 2021; Government of Canada, 2021). These antigens are then displayed on the surface of the cell, where immune cells in our immune system recognize them, commence an immune response, and begin making antibodies (Cao and Gao, 2021; Government of Canada, 2021). The mRNA is degraded after protein synthesis (Government of Canada, 2021). Antibodies recognize the spike protein on cells, block them to prevent further infection, and mark the cells for destruction (Corum and Zimmer, 2021). Antigen-presenting cells activate killer T cells to destroy cells displaying the spike protein on them (Corum and Zimmer, 2021). This teaches the body how to react defensively to SARS-CoV-2.

However, it is important to note that immunity is not immediate. Both the Pfizer and the Moderna vaccines require 2 doses for maximum protection, 21 days apart for Pfizer and one month apart for Moderna (Government of Canada, 2021). It takes approximately 2 weeks for significant immunity to develop. Trials with 30,000 participants showed that the Moderna vaccine was 94.1% effective in protecting participants from COVID-19 starting 2 weeks after the second dose was administered. For the Pfizer vaccine, trials with 40,000 participants showed that the vaccine was 95% effective in preventing COVID-19 in participants aged 16 and above and 100% effective in preventing COVID-19 in participants aged 12-15 years old starting 1 week after the second dose was administered (Polack et al., 2020; Government of Canada, 2021). The Pfizer vaccine is only approved for individuals who are aged 12 and older as efficacy and safety outcomes for those younger than 12 have not yet been evaluated (Government of Canada, 2021). The Moderna vaccine, on the other hand, is only approved for individuals who are aged 18 and older as efficacy and safety outcomes for those younger than 18 have not yet been evaluated.

For further context, mRNA vaccines have the ability to be rapidly developed, within days or months after sequencing the target virus, giving them an advantage over conventional vaccines which can take years to develop, research, and make effective (Cao and Gao, 2021). MRNA vaccines can also be quickly and inexpensively produced. Furthermore, because mRNA does not contain infectious viral elements, the vaccine risks are lower than with other conventional vaccines. However, this does not mean that these vaccines are completely free from side effects. Because vaccines trigger an immune response, their side effects are often similar to those felt during real infection - although they are generally milder and last a shorter amount of time (Oxford Vaccine Group, n.d.). In the clinical trials for the Pfizer vaccine, incidences of Bell's palsy, chills, fever, fatigue, and pain at the site of injection were reported (Cao and Gao, 2021). On the bright side, these are not uncommon or novel vaccine side effects and few serious adverse side effects were found (Government of Canada, 2021; Cao and Gao, 2021). However, the Pfizer website also reports that there is a very small chance of having a severe allergic reaction to the vaccine after receiving a dose, where signs may include difficulty breathing, swelling, a fast heartbeat, a rash, dizziness, or weakness. This may be because the Pfizer vaccine contains polyethylene glycol (PEG), which belongs to a group of known allergens commonly found in medicine (Oxford Vaccine Group, n.d.). Similar safety outcomes and risks have been established for the Moderna vaccine which also contains PEG as an ingredient (Government of Canada, 2021). Regardless, the development and approval of these novel vaccines within a year was unprecedented and a major victory for both the scientific community and everyone hoping for a quick end to the pandemic.

AstraZeneca and Janssen

The Janssen (Ad26.COV2.S) and AstraZeneca (ChAdOx1-S or AZD1222) COVID-19 vaccines are adenovirus vector vaccines. The Janssen vaccine was developed by a division of Johnson & Johnson Inc. called Janssen Pharmaceutica, a medical research and pharmaceutical company. The vaccine began development in January of 2020, and started clinical trials in July of 2020 (Corum and Zimmer, 2021). It was authorized for emergency use by the FDA on February 27, 2021. The AstraZeneca vaccine was actually made in collaboration with researchers at the University of Oxford in Oxford, England, who began development of the vaccine in January of 2020. AstraZeneca, a British and Swedish biotechnology and pharmaceutical company, only partnered with the researchers at Oxford on April 30th, 2020 after clinical trials had begun in order to help develop and distribute the vaccine. The vaccine was approved for use by Canada in February of 2021. As of June 13, 2021, the AstraZeneca vaccine has not yet been approved or authorized for emergency use in the United States by the FDA (Food and Drug Administration, n.d.).

This adenovirus vector form of vaccine is more traditional than the novel mRNA technology vaccines and has previously been used to combat Ebola, Middle East respiratory syndrome, and other diseases (Government of Canada, 2021; Jia et al., 2019). Adenoviruses are common viruses in humans and animals that can cause colds or other illnesses (Government of Canada, 2021). In vaccines, they serve as a delivery vehicle to the cell and are genetically modified so that they cannot replicate inside of our cells and cause illness (Government of Canada, 2021; Corum and Zimmer 2021). The AstraZeneca vaccine uses a modified chimpanzee adenovirus (Corum and Zimmer, 2021). Inside it, scientists add DNA which codes for the SARS-CoV-2 spike protein (Corum and Zimmer, 2021). When the vaccine is injected into the arm of an individual, the modified adenoviruses attach themselves onto the surface of cells and endocytosis occurs. They then travel to the nucleus of the cell and push their DNA inside, allowing the cell to transcribe it into mRNA and then translate it into spike proteins outside of the nucleus. Then, similar to the mRNA vaccines, the spike proteins are displayed on the surface of the cell, alerting the immune system and triggering an immune response to create antibodies. The adenovirus also helps to alert the cell and activate a strong immune response. The Janssen vaccine works similarly, but instead uses a human adenovirus (Government of Canada, 2021). As well, the Janssen vaccine only requires a single dose while the AstraZeneca vaccine requires two, 4-12 weeks apart..

Efficacy of the Janssen vaccine at preventing COVID-19 was found to be 66% starting 2 weeks after vaccination based on trials with approximately 43,000 participants (Government of Canada 2021). The AstraZeneca vaccine showed an efficacy of 62% starting 2 weeks after the second dose (Government of Canada, 2021). Both vaccines are only approved for individuals who are aged 18 or older, as efficacy and safety outcomes have not yet been fully evaluated for those under 18.

For the AstraZeneca vaccine, concerns about blood clotting have been raised. In March 2021, a number of European countries halted the administration of AstraZeneca after reports of vaccinated individuals experiencing thromboembolism came out. Specifically, 7 out of 20 million vaccinated individuals experienced disseminated intravascular coagulation (DIC) and 18 experienced cerebral venous sinus thrombosis (CVST) (European Medicines Agency, 2021). However, an analysis by Østergaard et al. (2021) found that the number of these cases did not differ from the normal rate and thus it was very possible that the incidences may have just been coincidence. As well, despite the possible link between the AstraZeneca vaccine and blood clots, the European Medicines Agency concluded that the benefits of vaccination outweigh any risks (European Medicines Agency, 2021). However, patients who have received the AstraZeneca vaccine should still be vigilant of thromboembolism symptoms such as severe headache, seizures, impaired vision, unusual pain, bleeding, blood blisters, swelling, redness, pallor, or coldness (Ontario Ministry of Health, 2021). Other side effects of the AstraZeneca vaccine included arm pain after injection, chills, fever, joint pain, muscle aches, fatigue, and headaches (Oxford Vaccine Group, n.d.). Side effects of the Janssen vaccine have been similar to those of AstraZeneca's (Government of Canada, 2021). Additionally, cases of fainting after individuals received the Janssen vaccine have been reported (Centers for Disease Control and Prevention, 2021). However, these cases were rare - only 653 out of nearly 8 million doses - and it is not yet evident whether the cause of the fainting was a direct result of the vaccine or other factors such as anxiety (Centers for Disease Control and Prevention, 2021).

The Pfizer vaccine must be stored at -80 °C and thus requires dry ice and special freezers for transportation (Cao and Gao, 2021; Centers for Disease Control and Prevention, 2021). Moderna requires storage at -20 °C (Cao and Gao, 2021). Once these vaccines are thawed and unfrozen, there is only a short window of time where they can be administered (Centers for Disease Control and Prevention, 2021). This is due to the fragility of RNA (Cao and Gao, 2021). In contrast, the AstraZeneca and Janssen vaccines, which use DNA and have protection from the durable protein coat of the adenovirus delivery vehicle, do not require special freezing and can be kept under normal refrigeration temperatures of 2 °C to 8° C (Corum and Zimmer, 2021; Santos et al., 2021). In fact, vials of the AstraZeneca vaccine, when unopened and refrigerated, are actually expected to last up to six months while the Janssen vaccine is expected to last up to three (Corum and Zimmer, 2021). This offers a huge advantage in terms of distribution. Places that may not have access to cold storage (such as rural and underdeveloped areas) can maintain and administer the adenovirus vaccines much more easily than the mRNA vaccines. As well, it was previously mentioned that the Pfizer and Moderna vaccines contain a known allergen, polyethylene glycol (PEG). The AstraZeneca and Janssen vaccines do not contain PEG and thus may potentially be offered as alternatives for those with severe allergies (Government of Canada, 2021; Oxford Vaccine Group, n.d.). However, the AstraZeneca and Janssen vaccines do contain polysorbate 80, which may in some rare cases cause type I hypersensitivity reactions (Ontario Ministry of Health, 2021).

Although these vaccines were made to combat the pandemic, our world still faces another major threat - the climate crisis. Now more than ever, the environmental impact of every action must be considered and evaluated. With an initiative as large as manufacturing billions of vaccines to inoculate the global population, it is crucial that the influence on the environment does not go ignored. The special storage requirements of the Pfizer and Moderna vaccines give them direct total equivalent warming impacts (TEWI) of 4111.99 kg CO_2 and 876.97 kg CO_2, respectively (Santos et al., 2021). TEWI is a measure of contribution to global warming. In contrast, the direct TEWIs due to the storage requirements of the AstraZeneca and Janssen vaccines are 598.45 kg CO_2 each. To better understand this difference, the environmental impact of the storage requirements of the vaccines in the United States can be compared to CO_2 emissions of cars running 20,000 km. For the same number of doses, the Pfizer vaccine would have CO_2 emissions equivalent to 158,636.80 cars, the Moderna vaccine would have CO_2 emissions equivalent to 41,299.09 cars, and the AstraZeneca and Janssen vaccines would have CO_2 emissions equivalent to 17,279,32 cars each. Thus, the environmental impact of the former two vaccines is immensely greater. As well, it is important to note that because the Janssen vaccine only requires one dose unlike the other vaccines, it actually has the lowest environmental impact in reality. These differences could be an important factor for nations to consider when trying to achieve sustainability alongside their vaccine rollouts. Overall, despite their lower efficacy when compared to the Pfizer and Moderna vaccines, the AstraZeneca and Janssen vaccines offer unique advantages that will contribute greatly to protecting and maintaining our global health.

CoronaVac
CoronaVac is an inactivated vaccine. As discussed in Chapter
2, this means that the vaccine uses killed microorganisms.
Developed by Sinovac, a private Chinese pharmaceutical
company, it began development in January of 2020 and was
given conditional approval for use in China on February
6, 2021 (Corum and Zimmer, 2021). To create the vaccine,
researchers obtained coronavirus samples from infected
patients and let them propagate in monkey kidney cells.
They then modified the viruses by covering them in an
inactivating reagent called beta-propiolactone to stop them
from replicating. By inactivating and killing the viruses,
they could now be injected into the human body without
causing COVID-19. However, antigen-presenting cells in the
body would still recognize and swallow them, activating an
immune response and allowing for the creation of antibodies.
Thus, the body could learn how to defend against live SARS-
CoV-2. Indeed, a clinical trial by Wu et al. (2021) showed
that compared to placebo groups, those administered
the vaccine showed considerable antibody development.
However, efficacy data has been mixed so far, with some
researchers finding the vaccine 91% effective at preventing
the development of severe COVID-19 and others only finding
a 50% effectiveness (Corum and Zimmer, 2021; Mallapaty,
2021). With regard to side effects, CoronaVac was found to
be safe with the most common side effects remaining mild
to moderate, such as headaches (Wu et al., 2021; Mallapaty,
2021). Similar to the AstraZeneca and Janssen vaccines,
the CoronaVac vaccine does not require special freezers
for storage, but instead can be kept in normal refrigeration
temperatures (2 °C to 8 °C) (Santos et al., 2021). Due to this,

the environmental impact of CoronaVac is also similar to the AstraZeneca and Janssen vaccines. It has also been reported that the vaccine can be expected to remain viable for up to three years under refrigeration.

Novavax

Novavax, Inc. is an American biotechnology company that develops vaccines in order to combat and prevent serious infectious diseases (Novavax, n.d.). They have previously worked to create vaccines for infectious diseases including Ebola, influenza, respiratory syncytial virus (RSV), Middle East respiratory syndrome (MERS), and severe acute respiratory syndrome (SARS). Despite this, the company is small and has been unable to bring any vaccines to market (Wadman 2020). In January of 2020, Novavax, Inc. began working on their NVX-CoV2373 vaccine for COVID-19 (Corum and Zimmer, 2021). NVX-CoV2373 is a protein subunit vaccine which has not yet filed for Emergency Use Authorization with the FDA or been approved in Canada despite showing very promising results from clinical trials. Protein-based vaccines are known to be a more traditional, proven form of vaccine compared to the novel mRNA-based vaccines. The hepatitis B vaccine which is usually one of the first vaccines administered to newborns is a protein-based vaccine (Wadman 2020). Indeed, against wild-type SARS-CoV-2, the Novavax vaccine has shown an efficacy rate of 96% (Corum and Zimmer, 2021). The vaccine has also shown high promise for protecting against variants, with an efficacy rate of 86% against the 501Y.V1 (B.1.1.7) United Kingdom variant and 49% against the 501Y.V2 (B.1.351) South African variant (Corum and Zimmer, 2021).

Researchers at Novavax created the vaccine by inserting

a modified spike protein gene into a baculovirus and then infecting moth cells with the virus in order to grow and harvest spikes from the cell membranes of the moth cells (Corum and Zimmer, 2021). The spikes were then assembled into nanoparticles which resembled the structure of SARS-CoV-2, although these nanoparticles would not be able to replicate or cause COVID-19 (Corum and Zimmer, 2021). Each nanoparticle is 30 to 40 nanometers in diameter and contains up to 14 spike proteins (Wadman 2020). Then, the nanoparticles along with saponin, a soap bark tree compound, are injected intramuscularly into the upper arm (Corum and Zimmer, 2021; Wadman 2020). The soapbark tree compound is an adjuvant that works to attract immune cells to the site of injection and activates a stronger response towards the foreign nanoparticles (Corum and Zimmer, 2021). Antigen-presenting cells swallow the nanoparticles and provoke an immune response where the body creates antibodies that can block SARS-CoV-2 spike proteins and is thus able to defend against infection, similar to the vaccines discussed previously (Corum and Zimmer, 2021). The Novavax vaccine is also expected to be stable for weeks when kept under normal refrigeration temperatures of 2°C to 8°C (Wadman 2020).

Distribution and Vaccine Inequity

As mentioned in the introduction of this chapter, for the COVID-19 pandemic to end, the global population must reach herd immunity where an estimated 70% of the population must be vaccinated. For this to occur, distribution of the vaccines must be equitable. However, this has not been the case so far. According to Rouw et al. (2021), high income countries collectively own over half (54% or 4.6 billion) of all COVID-19 vaccine doses, despite only constituting 19% of the global adult population. The number of doses purchased are far greater than needed. According to Fontanent et al. (2021), the number has sometimes been close to 9 doses per person. In contrast, low-middle income countries and nations only hold a collective 670 million doses (BBC News, 2021). The Director General of WHO, Tedros Adhanom Ghebreyesus, reported that in high income countries, nearly one in four people have been vaccinated against COVID-19. However, in low income countries, this number is only one in approximately five-hundred people. While high income countries have enough doses to vaccinate their entire adult populations more than two times over, the low and middle income countries only have enough to vaccinate approximately one-third of theirs (Roux et al., 2021). Unless the countries which have been hoarding vaccine doses redistribute them somehow (perhaps through donation), or unless support for vaccine production increases, the entire global population will not be able to be inoculated (Rouw et al. 2021). According to Roux et al. (2021), some high income countries such as France, the United States, Norway, and the United Kingdom have indeed indicated their intention to donate excess doses.

Luckily, COVAX, an initiative led by the Coalition for Epidemic Preparedness Innovations (CEPI), Gavi, the Vaccine Alliance, UNICEF, and the World Health Organization (WHO) involving 190 governments (90% of the global population) has been created in order to combat these inequities (Roux et al., 2021). Specifically, the goal of this initiative has been to distribute 2 billion doses of COVID-19 vaccines to those who are most vulnerable by the end of 2021. The allocation of these vaccines is being laid out by WHO. Indeed, COVAX has purchased 1.2 billion doses (13% of the total COVID-19 vaccine doses). As of June 17th, 2021, 88 million doses have been distributed to 131 participants (Gavi, the Vaccine Alliance, 2021). Vulnerable countries such as Nepal, Ethiopia, Colombia, Afghanistan, Ukraine, and The Philippines are a few of many that have received doses through the initiative. However, COVAX faces a massive funding gap of 7.2 billion USD for 2021 (Roux et al., 2021). As well, even with all of the COVAX doses distributed, low and middle income countries would only be able to vaccinate approximately half of their adult populations. Based on the total number of vaccine doses purchased, these low and middle income countries should have been able to vaccinate 86% of their adult populations if it had not been for the stockpiling of higher income countries. This fact truly allows one to grasp the magnitude of vaccine disparity. The equitable distribution of vaccines is in the best interest of all, as failure to reach herd immunity will result in major economic consequences for high-income countries that could have been avoided with the curbing of the pandemic.

Vaccine distribution has also been inequitable on a smaller scale. Even within the high income countries, vaccines have been disproportionately administered. Many countries had vaccine rollout plans which included determining which populations were most at risk for severe COVID-19 and then vaccinating those individuals first. The UK Joint Committee prioritized the following risk groups: residents and staff in care homes for older adults, frontline health and social care workers, those aged 65 and older, and other at-risk groups. Although rollout plans such as this seem simple and fair enough at first glance, a lack of attention to specific challenges some individuals face has led to disparity (Jean-Jacques and Bauchner 2021). In the United States, pharmacy deserts have created a great challenge for some people hoping to get vaccinated. The Rural Policy Research Institute conducted an analysis which found that 111 rural counties in the United States actually had no pharmacy able to administer vaccines (Hawryluk and Kaiser Health News 2021). This meant that residents of these areas would have to travel great distances in order to receive a vaccination - something that might not be possible for everyone (Hawryluk and Kaiser Health News 2021). Indeed, residents of rural areas had lower vaccine coverage (38.9%) than residents of urban areas (45.7%) based on reports from CDC researchers from December 14th, 2020 to April 10th, 2021 (Beusekom 2021). Furthermore, a vaccine class gap also exists. A survey conducted in April 2021 of over 2000 adults showed that non-college graduates were much less likely to have been vaccinated and had more distrust in the vaccines (Leonhardt 2021). Jean-Jacques and Bauchner (2021) suggest that vaccine disparities such as these may be narrowed by the following:

1. Prioritize vaccine distribution to zip codes that have been most severely affected by COVID-19 and that have high indexes of economic hardship.

2. Partner with local health care institutions, community organizations, and other trusted sources to promote vaccine awareness and uptake within local communities, with particular attention to institutions and organizations that serve communities who have borne the brunt of COVID-19 exposure, illness, and death.

3. Prioritize vaccine distribution to those who face mobility or other transportation barriers to receipt of the vaccine (eg, vans to deliver vaccine to homebound older persons, vaccination sites that are near public transportation, and hours of operation that are accessible to those who work or who rely on those who work during standard business hours).

4. Simplify registration procedures. Ensure registration options that do not require the internet or digital platforms (such as phone or in-person registration). Ensure registration is accessible to those with limited English proficiency or limited literacy. Registration should not require nonessential documentation, such as proof of citizenship, that is likely to deter individuals from immigrant communities from seeking vaccination. Offer vaccination options that do not require preregistration (eg, at local community centers, schools, houses of worship, or other highly frequented and trusted sites in the community) (para. 3).

Hopefully, by removing such barriers, vaccine inequities can be conquered and the COVID-19 pandemic can come to a swift end, not just for high income countries, but for all.

Efficacy for Older Adults

As mentioned in chapter 4, immunosenescence is associated with a decline in vaccine efficacy. The high-risk of older adults against COVID-19 is why this group among other vulnerable populations has been given vaccination priority. However, concerns about the efficacy of vaccines in older adults have been raised as previous research has shown that immunosenescence diminishes vaccine responses in the elderly. The influenza vaccination has been found to have an efficacy of only 30-40% in vulnerable older adults (Cox et al., 2020). However, results from COVID-19 vaccination clinical trials for older adults have been surprising and promising. In adults aged 70 and older, one dose of the Pfizer-BioNTech vaccine had an efficacy of 57-61% in the prevention of COVID-19 and one dose of the AstraZeneca vaccine had an efficacy of 60-73% (Beusekom, 2021). Utilizing the method of boosting – administering a second dose of the vaccine in order to further increase immunity against an antigen – increased the efficacy of Pfizer to 85-90% (Beusekom, 2021). Despite these encouraging results, data has still shown that compared to younger individuals, older adults are experiencing a reduced antibody response to the COVID-19 vaccines (Soize et al., 2020).

However, some methods exist for increasing the efficacy of vaccines and countering the effects of immunosenescence. Along with boosting, higher-dose vaccines and alternative routes of administration (ie. mucosal, oral) have shown potential for increasing vaccine efficacy (Aiello et al., 2019; Zhang et al,. 2016). As well, taking preventative measures such as maintaining proper nutrition and exercising can counteract the effects of immunosenescence (Aiello et al., 2019; Lord, 2013). Proper nutrition will also protect against zinc deficiency, something that can be harmful as zinc has been linked with benefiting the immune system (Mocchegiani et al., 2006). Whole thymic transplantation is another intervention that has been explored as a way to restore immune function by increasing the number of naïve T cells and shown promising results (Aiello et al., 2019). Another identified potential future strategy is rooted in cellular and genetic therapy, where immune system cells may be rejuvenated through telomere elongation (Aiello et al., 2019). Currently, older adults have often been excluded from experimental drug trials, but the COVID-19 pandemic has propelled interest in this area forward (Cox et al. 2020; Pawelec and McElhaney 2021). Hopefully, in coming years, more research will be inclusive of older adults and work to find solutions for the restoration of immune function. Until then, older adults should remain reassured by the fact that they still benefit greatly from vaccination versus remaining unvaccinated and should receive COVID-19 vaccines when given the chance (Centers for Disease Control and Prevention, 2021).

Variants and Vaccination

Because many of the COVID-19 vaccine projects were launched before the identification of new SARS-CoV-2 variants, concerns have been raised about the efficacy of vaccines against them. How effective are the current vaccines against different variants? Could the virus mutate to escape the vaccine? Novavax included data in their studies that showed high efficacy against the variants, but what about the other vaccines? In October of 2020, WHO reported that because the vaccines induce a broad immune response, it is likely that they will still be effective against variants to some degree. Indeed, recent studies involving the Pfizer and Moderna vaccines have reported this. A analysis published in the New England Journal of Medicine by Abu-Raddad et al. (2021) reported that the Pfizer vaccine had an approximate efficacy of 87.0% to 89.5% for protecting against the 501Y. V1 (B.1.1.7) variant and 72.1% to 75.0% for the 501Y.V2 (B.1.351) variant based on data from Qatar. Moderna Inc. has reported that an additional booster shot of their current COVID-19 vaccine has been shown to increase protection against the 501Y.V2 (B.1.351) and P.1 variants (O'Donnell, 2021). Similarly, an analysis by Public Health England found that the AstraZeneca vaccine offers a protection of more than

90% against hospitalization from COVID-19 caused by the
B.1.617.2 Delta variant (Burger and Nair, 2021). More studies
and trials are currently underway to determine the exact
clinical efficacies of vaccines, modifications, and booster shots
against the variants (France-Presse, 2021; O'Donnell, 2021) .

According to Darby and Hiscox (2021), the risk of the virus
mutating further to escape immunity is hard to predict.
Although the current vaccines provide protection against
the dominant SARS-CoV-2 variants (which are still in close
genetic proximity to the wild-type CoV), it is probable that as
the virus mutates further and variants diverge, vaccines will
need to be modified and updated (Darby and Hiscox, 2021).
Indeed, Moderna Inc. and AstraZeneca have been developing
and testing new experimental vaccines to further protect
against the variants. As well, as mentioned in chapter 4,
the longer the virus is around, the more it is able to mutate.
Although it may seem like the pandemic is coming to an end
for those in high income countries, other areas will not be
so quick to vaccinate their populations (Darby and Hiscox,
2021). Thus, it is imperative to realize that SARS-CoV-2 and its
variants are not going to stop mutating or disappear any time
soon and the goal of global inoculation will have to consider
this challenge (Darby and Hiscox, 2021).

Long-Term Immunity?
Due to the novelty of these vaccines, long-term immunity
is still a huge unknown. It may be possible that months
after receiving the vaccination, the immune response
will diminish (Corum and Zimmer, 2021). It may also be
possible that memory B cells and memory T cells will retain
information on how to defend against SARS-CoV-2 for years
to come (Corum and Zimmer, 2021). In the case of waning

immunity, an additional booster shot may be administered within 12 months of the second dose in order to heighten protection once again - especially for older adults who face the challenges of immunosenescence (Baraniuk, 2021). As it stands, researchers continue to monitor the effects of the vaccine and will closely do so for the upcoming few years.

Limitations

Despite many countries making progress with their vaccination campaigns, many challenges still stand in the way of complete global inoculation against COVID-19. Along with the difficulties associated with vaccine rollout and equity, another big obstacle that will be explored in upcoming chapters is vaccine hesitancy. An additional challenge is the possibility of the virus transferring to new reservoir host populations and spilling back over into the human population (Richman, 2021). Because of this, unlike SARS-CoV-1, it is very unlikely that SARS-CoV-2 will be completely eradicated. As mentioned previously, this also creates a threat of variants evolving to escape the vaccines. Thus, it is important to keep in mind the limitations of the vaccines and understand the importance of maintaining public health measures and guidelines. These measures may include limiting contact with others, covering coughs, sneezing into elbows, sanitizing and washing hands frequently, remaining at least 1 metre away from others, avoiding crowds, wearing a face mask, and keeping rooms properly ventilated (World Health Organization, 2020). Vaccines are an incredibly powerful, effective tool of modern medicine, but they do not make us invulnerable.

Chapter 6: The Search For a Preventive for COVID-19

Following the World Health Organization's confirmation of COVID-19 cases in China, Thailand, Italy, and eventually, on a global scale, the medical community fixated on discovering a cure (WHO, 2020). With the virus being novel, meaning unknown, two streams of thought naturally emerged in preventive discussions: Some scientists proposed a vaccine specific to the virus, while others contemplated repurposing existing vaccines and medications (Billingsley, 2020). In this chapter, we will be discussing the existing medications evaluated for prevention, how medications were identified through ligand-based screening, and the nuances between vaccines and medications. Through this discussion, we will obtain a greater understanding of the development of conventional medicines and vaccines and of their role in treatment. To begin, we'll start with hydroxychloroquine as it bred havoc and confusion after being coined as the first medication showing promise in laboratory settings (WebMD, 2021).

Hydroxychloroquine
Sandhu (2020) defines hydroxychloroquine, also known as oral Plaquenil, as a "disease-modifying antirheumatic drug" (para. 1). Hydroxychloroquine, a drug first discovered in the 1940s, was initially used to ward off and treat malaria caused by the Anopheles gambiae mosquito, a whining, blackish-brown insect with elongated palps and that's

notorious for transmitting infected blood (Sandhu, 2020; Orkin, 2021). The drug, today, has branched out in its uses, alleviating everything from rheumatoid arthritis, to lupus symptoms, and other autoimmune diseases. It is unclear why hydroxychloroquine has remedied malaria and the symptoms of autoimmune diseases for several decades now. Many researchers believe the drug works as it "interferes with the communication of cells in the immune system" (Sandhu. 2020, para. 1). It would be safe to induce that recent testing during the COVID-19 pandemic has likely enriched our understanding of the drug and its uses.

Testing Hydroxychloroquine as a Treatment for COVID-19
In April of 2020, the beginning months of the pandemic for the majority of countries, practitioners debated over hydroxychloroquine and its preventive abilities, especially after the fervent touting from former American President Donald Trump (Facher, 2020). As you likely remember, rousing discussions and the testing of hydroxychloroquine snowballed from that point out.

How did the kerfuffle begin though? Upon President Trump receiving a letter from a Westchester Country doctor detailing the efficacy of hydroxychloroquine against COVID-19, he encouraged Americans to discuss taking the drug with their doctor (Sommerfeldt, 2020). The antibiotic, azithromycin (also known as Z-Pak or Zithromax), which often treats bacterial infections in the ears, lungs, and organs, was to be ingested with hydroxychloroquine to aid in the drug's efficacy (Llamas, 2020; Facher, 2020). To support his recommendation of temporarily using the drugs, the former president mentioned a small but successful study performed by a group of French doctors, one of which included the controversial researcher Didier Raoult, who is well-known and now questioned for his star-crossed love for hydroxychloroquine. The French study has since been scrutinized for its science and for its failure to randomize its sampling (Facher, 2020). In the weeks following Trump's announcement from the White House podium, the amount of hydroxychloroquine prescribed surpassed the country's stockpile (Facher, 2020). Unaware of the many forms of the drug and feeling confident in its preventive abilities, some Americans skipped the doctor's visit and resorted to self-medicating chloroquine phosphate, an FDA unregulated, intensified form of the drug, designed for cleaning aquariums and fish tanks (Shepherd, 2020). Additionally, from surges in demand for hydroxychloroquine, lupus patients were unable to refill their prescriptions. To provide context, 31 million doses of hydroxychloroquine sulfate were donated by the pharmaceutical companies Sandoz and Bayer around this time (Facher, 2020). That figure alludes to the vast number of Americans depending on the drug, all in the hopes of protecting themselves from the coronavirus.

Some snails crossing the front lawn later (meaning, after weeks and months of testing hydroxychloroquine), officials were more definite about whether or not the drug was COVID-19's solution. A warning, the results weren't substantial. Conducting a series of small tests, scientists concluded that hydroxychloroquine exhibited mixed results (WebMD, 2021). As mentioned earlier, one study in France demonstrated that hydroxychloroquine reduced the amount of the COVID-19 virus in patients, but another study in China found patients failed to "benefit substantially compared to patients who did not use it" (Facher, 2020, para. 12). One finding alerted the FDA though, leading the organization to completely retract temporary emergency approval (WebMD, 2020). In addition to retracting use, the FDA cautioned against prescribing hydroxychloroquine since it could cause cardiotoxicity or heart damage, albeit on rare occasions (WebMD, 2020; Facher, 2020). More relative to diminishing the virus, the FDA retracted approval because the drug was found ineffective in preventing COVID-related deaths or illnesses (WebMD, 2020). Health officials now warn that taking the drug while battling a severe case of the virus could be fatal for those with existing heart conditions or with co-morbidities (Facher, 2020).

Practitioners' Doubts for Hydroxychloroquine
As you may remember during the March and April news hysteria in 2020, few health practitioners seemed to promote or be optimistic about hydroxychloroquine. In fact, many doctors surmised hydroxychloroquine was not the cure even before additional hydroxychloroquine studies were conducted and before the media was blown into a Trump frenzy (Facher, 2020). Countless practitioners reported they were unconvinced of the drug's preventive abilities because of this one simple observation: lupus and arthritis patients, who were already routinely taking hydroxychloroquine, were frequently being diagnosed with COVID-19.

It may appear contradictory, but, today, scientists are still intrigued by and support efforts to study chloroquine. Early studies of hydroxychloroquine bubbled with promise as the drug showed an antiviral effect on infected SARS-CoV-2 cells (WebMD, 2021). Its resistance to the virus only went so far though. While the drug had demonstrated an impeccable resistance to COVID-19 in laboratory settings, the results failed to be replicated in people or real-life situations. Upon the FDA realizing its inability to protect people, the testing of hydroxychloroquine was eventually discontinued by the administration. That wouldn't speak for other scientists, as we'll see.

It is important to note that around this time, besides hydroxychloroquine, an array of drugs and natural remedies were being evaluated for their therapeutic abilities, including garlic, blood pressure pills, and even alcohol (World Health Organization, 2020). Of course, alcohol, for one, was known to cause health problems and to weaken the body's immunity to pathogens (NIAAA, 2020). To say the least, health officials were quick to evaluate natural alternatives, knowing consumers were buying excessive amounts of them in hopes of strengthening their immune systems. Soon, we'll discuss some of the other medications that underwent a closer look by scientists through rigorous testing and study.

Why Were Existing Medications and Vaccines Considered?

> *"Think of it as a whack-a-mole game. Instead of having one hammer, you have two hammers, which is more effective. We're trying to give the scientific community two hammers instead of one" (Huzar, 2020, "Three Drugs Identified").*

Examining the logistics and the extent of the global health crisis guided scientists in their decision-making. Upon scientists pondering all the detrimental factors, such as the costs of developing a vaccine, the duress of lockdowns, the likelihood of an endemic, the cultural effects of isolation, and the seriousness of COVID-19, repurposing a former vaccine or medication became viewed as a time worth spent, especially if it worked or, better yet, saved lives (Huzar, 2020). While scientists worked on developing a COVID-19 vaccine, some would, alternatively, study previous vaccines and medications to see if they could be repurposed for treatment. Aside from the concerns already listed, a major influencing factor behind studying former medicines was the issue of time. As stated by Huzar (2020):

> *According to a report in The Lancet, on average, vaccines take 10 years to develop (some sources say even 12-15 years). Even with experts greatly accelerating research due to the urgency of the global pandemic, the report notes that an initial vaccine may take more than 18 months to be developed, manufactured, and distributed to people around the world. (para. 7)*

Once scientists reflected on the virus' nature and the time required to safely develop and produce a vaccine, repurposing medications or a vaccine proved a constructive step in emergency action. As much as the pursuit was time and cost-effective, however, scientists were continuously met by a thwart in their studies—medications, such as remdesivir, an Ebola treatment, and hydroxychloroquine were found effective against COVID-19 in test tubes, but ineffective in real life (Huzar, 2020). Environmental influences played a larger role than anticipated. To researchers, it felt a breakthrough was almost tangible but not quite. How were scientists to replicate their findings, a resistance to COVID-19, in an imperfect, disrupted setting? After all, it would be beneficial if the world had medicine to treat those sick with COVID-19. It was the equivalent of two hammers, not just one.

The Nuances and Role of Conventional Medicines and Vaccines

The intention behind making vaccines and conventional medicines greatly differ. To elaborate, vaccines, which are increasingly complicated and time-consuming, are intended for "persons not yet exhibiting disease symptoms to prevent the occurrence of disease" (Calina et al., 2020, p. 2). As best described by Accra (2015), vaccines are "a [biological] product that stimulates a person's immune system to produce immunity to a specific disease, protecting the person from that disease" (p. 4). A biological product refers to something of large, complex molecules, sometimes "produced through biotechnology in a living system, such as a microorganism, plant cell, or animal cell" (FDA, n.d., p. 2). Vaccines which are "usually administered through needle injections, can be administered by mouth or sprayed into the nose" (Accra, 2015, p. 4).

Conventional medicines, which are of a chemical, biological, or herbal product, are geared towards "the treatment of a disease whose symptoms have emerged" (Calina et al., 2020; Accra, 2015, p. 10). Medications are given to "treat, diagnose, or prevent disease" for the benefit of an individual, not for a group of people or herd immunity (Accra, 2015, p. 21). Most chemical drugs are consumed orally through tablets, capsules, suspensions, but some are administered via other routes, including intravenous (IV), subcutaneous injections (SI), dermally, and intramuscular injection (IM). Unlike vaccines which require cold storage, medications withstand warmer and fluctuating temperatures. Although they appear oppositional, medicines and vaccines share similarities in efficacy, safety, and quality standards, and in their ability to cause adverse events or to interact with disease, drugs, and other vaccines (Accra, 2015).

In summary, different frames of thinking and approaches are required in the development of medicines and vaccines. Their main difference stems from how medicines are treatments and vaccines are preventives. It can be helpful for later recall to think of how both are administered at different times. But, now that we touched on the key differences between medicines and vaccines, as well as the intended role of prescription drugs during the COVID crisis, let's discuss how the medications were selected. Later, we will explore the three medications found effective against the virus in test tubes.

Virtually Screening Medications for Potentiality
Virtual screening is used in the "drug discovery process for lead identification, lead optimization, and scaffold hopping" (Hamza et al., 2013, p. 1). The virtual screening method, which is used to discover new drugs, is an inexpensive, relatively fast alternative to high-throughput screenings.

Oftentimes, medications are identified through high throughput screening (HTS), which "involves automating the testing of many different medications ... [and] then analyzing the results with a computer" (Huzar, 2020, para. 14). Some issues with HTS screening alarmed scientists though. After some studies highlighted issues in HTS's reliability and accuracy, Lancet scientists and other researchers, who were testing hydroxychloroquine-related medications for their efficacy against COVID-19, adapted a ligand-based virtual screening (LBVS) approach. Adapting the LBVS approach, the scientists' scan thus focused on medications with properties akin to hydroxychloroquine (Huzar, 2020). As mentioned earlier, scientists continued studying the therapeutic as it exhibited the most promising results in laboratories (Balfour, 2020).

According to Hamza et al. (2013), "ligand-based virtual screening methods use the information present in known active ligands rather than the structure of a target protein for both lead identification and optimization" (p. 1). To single in on known active ligands via scanning enables researchers to measure the similarities between ligands and to collect their reliability scoring. Meaning, scientists were able to identify similar hydroxychloroquine treatments through the ligand approach.

Amodiaquine

Studying roughly 4,000 drugs through LBVS scanning, scientists pinpointed three drugs that potentially prevented COVID-19 (Huzar, 2020). One of them was amodiaquine. As defined by the U.S. National Library of Medicine (NIH) (2017), amodiaquine, "is a synthetic aminoquinoline that acts by binding to the protozoal or parasitic DNA and preventing DNA and RNA production and subsequent protein synthesis" (p. 1). Figuratively speaking, amodiaquine is like a first cousin to chloroquine, as its structure is relative to it. Amodiaquine is recognized as "a useful agent for falciparum malaria, but because of its potential for causing hepatotoxicity, it is no longer used for antimalarial prophylaxis" (NIH, 2017, p. 1). Scientists hypothesize that if amodiaquine was mixed with remdesivir or favipiravir, the combination would result in an effective preventive. As we know, the drug's efficacy could only be reproduced in laboratory settings, but scientists persist that the drugs are worth studying further in clinical trials (Huzar, 2020).

Zuclopenthixol

The second drug scientists identified was zuclopenthixol (Huzar, 2020). Often in the form of a liquid, zuclopenthixol, also known as zuclopenthixol or zuclopenthixolum, is an antipsychotic drug that balances chemical substances in the brain, reducing the symptoms of schizophrenia (National Center for Biotechnology Information, 2021; Stewart, 2018). Scientists hypothesized that combining zuclopenthixol with remesivir, a 2014 Ebola drug, or with favipiravir, an antimalarial medicine, may be "particularly effective" (Huzar, 2020). Again, efficacy could not be replicated in environments outside of the laboratory.

Nebivolol

The third and last therapeutic identified was nebivolol (Huzar, 2020). Nebivolol, of the class of medications called beta-blockers, is used to treat high blood pressure. The medication "works by relaxing blood vessels and slowing heart rate to improve blood flow and decrease blood pressure" (U.S. National Library of Medicine, 2021, para. 1). At the University of Tennessee Health Science Center, where scientists conducted in vitro experiments, which are tests inside of a laboratory, they discovered that nebivolol blocked against the SARS-2 virus—but, of course, only within that limited, confined setting (Balfour, 2020). The researchers also concluded that the adjuvant remdesivir, a substance to assist the immune system in generating antibodies, would increase its overall efficacy (Balfour, 2020; Moore, 2021).

All of the three drugs discussed are what scientists refer to as "promising candidates," and they have plans to study the therapeutics further in clinical studies (Balfour, 2020). To date, a preventive, one that could assist or treat those bedridden or suffering from the short and long-term effects of COVID-19, hasn't been discovered yet. Until then, scientists will continue searching for a preventive measure.

Chapter 7: The Business Behind The Vaccines

With the growing need for better and more effective vaccines, traditional vaccine companies are adapting by increasing their manufacturing capacity and innovative ability. Vaccine manufacturing has changed drastically over the past 30 years. In 1980, the introduction of good manufacturing practices to vaccine production, caused manufacturing costs to increase and profit margins to decrease (Sheridan, 2005).The vaccine industry includes companies that are involved in the research, development, manufacturing, sales, marketing, and distribution of vaccines. These companies receive their revenue primarily from the sale of vaccines. The vaccine industry is small compared to the pharmaceutical industry, but growing. In fact, Mercer Management consulting estimates the global market for both childhood and adult vaccines has grown approximately 10 percent per year since 1992 (Institute of Medicine, 2003).

Vaccine Market Structure
There are typically two types of vaccine markets. The first is the price taker markets, generally seen in domestic markets and characterized by export (procurement agencies), many suppliers and competition. In this type of market, there are stable prices and lower research & development (R&D) costs due to transfer of technology. Therefore, these markets have low barriers to entry.

The other type of vaccine market that can occur are monopoly markets. These markets generally arise from novel vaccines and are characterized by having a few suppliers that have the ability to set the price of vaccines. In general, monopoly markets have higher prices due to their high R&D costs and risks.

Vaccine companies are found in 50 different countries, but the largest companies are primarily located in the United States or Europe (Douglas & Samant, 2018). Vaccine manufacturing is concentrated in four manufactures (GSK, Pfizer, Merck, and Sanofi) and they control 90% of global vaccine value (World Health Organization [WHO], 2020). The companies SII, GSK, Sanofi, BBIL, and Haffkine together produce 60% of the global volume of vaccines. The United States and European based companies have the dominant share of vaccine business on a revenue basis. The mid-sized manufacturers are mainly located in Asia and compete in regional and new vaccine markets and are gradually growing their market share. They offer additional and often more affordable choices (WHO, 2020).

Manufacturing vaccines is one of the most challenging industries (Plotkin et al., 2017). The most basic manufacturing steps to consistently produce safe and effective vaccines over the course of the vaccine life cycle can be difficult to execute (Plotkin et al., 2017). Complications can arise from the near infinite combinations of biological variability in basic starting materials, the microorganism itself, the microbial culture's environmental condition, and during the multiple steps in the purification process. Additionally, the methods used to analyze biological processes and antigens during vaccine production have high inherent variability. Failure to manage these risks can result in costly product recalls and suspensions which could result in further fines and penalties if the manufacturer is unable to fulfill supply agreements. In the broader scope, lack of vaccine supply can disrupt immunization programs and negatively impact national public health outcomes (Plotkin et al., 2017). Manufacturers also need to have their vaccine production process licensed by regulatory authorities. Process changes, regardless of how subtle, may alter the final product's purity, safety, or efficacy which may not be detected by in vitro analytics. Therefore, a new clinical trial may be required in order for the manufacturer to maintain their product licence. A high proportion of vaccine manufacturers fail due to the mismanaging the compounded risk of biological and physical variability. This is also why the number of vaccine manufacturers remains low, despite the unmet demand of vaccines around the world.

Cost Structure
There are a lot of costs associated with the manufacturing and distribution of vaccines. The cost structure for a vaccine manufacturer can be broken down into four major components: fixed costs, variable costs, indirect costs, and regulatory, licensing, and commercialization costs
In general, fixed costs are the most significant hurdle for vaccine manufacturers. The large initial investment required acts as a high barrier to entry in the vaccine market. The manufacturing facilities, including all the machinery and the land its on, represent a major fixed cost to manufacturers. Additionally, the ongoing maintenance, including repairs, upkeep, and utilities, are another significant cost to manufacturers. This initial investment can range anywhere between 50 million to 700 million USD. For example, Pfizer

spent a total of 600 million USD over five years to build their manufacturing site in the United States (Plotkin et al., 2017). The design of manufacturing facilities is extremely important. Manufacturers focus on utilizing the space as optimally as possible. They will force fit new processes with existing and established platforms to reduce the need for new facilities which would incur further costs to the company. This means a single piece of equipment in a facility could be used to make multiple different vaccines. Vaccine manufacturers are constantly innovating ways to force fit new processes in order to reduce their massive fixed costs.

Manufacturers will conduct extensive market research in order to properly allocate facility capacity to meet market demand. If the manufacturer miscalculates and the capacity is too low, then there could be a lack of supply and increased opportunity costs to the company. Opportunity cost refers to the potential benefits a company or individual misses out on by choosing one alternative over another. In this case, the opportunity cost would be the missed vaccine revenue due to not having enough capacity to meet the vaccine demand. Conversely, if the manufacturer overestimates demand and the capacity is too large, then the average fixed cost burden will increase per dose. The average fixed cost is calculated by dividing the high fixed costs over many doses. To reduce their average fixed costs, vaccine manufacturers will attempt to increase their production outputs. This is known as economies of scale, which is extremely advantageous to companies. Economies of scale will significantly decrease total fixed costs per dose as production volume increases.

Some companies have shifted their production towards multi-dose over single dose vials which simultaneously increase their production volume while reducing their filling costs. Economies of scale and reducing the average fixed costs is not something that happens overnight and can sometimes take years to achieve. Some manufacturing companies may need to develop a large vaccine portfolio before they can start to see a significant impact on their production costs.

Variable costs are expenses that vary with the level of production output. This can range from the amount of biological agents, vials and seals, packaging, shipping and import fees, and quality control testing kits used. In most cases, the biological agents are produced through complex biological production processes such as from yeast extracts, natural enzymes, or recombinant enzymes (Plotkin et al., 2017). However, these specialized raw materials might be limited in supply and subject to shortages if the demand is greater than the supplier's maximum output. Supply shortages of raw material can lead to manufacturers not meeting their vaccine quota which can lead to significant fines and loss of revenue. For a vaccine manufacturer, the cost of consumables are dependent on the normal dynamics of supply and demand. Biological material in low supply is generally more expensive. Additionally, the inherent biological variability in the raw material of animal origin requires vaccine manufacturers to extensively test and screen the samples for viral and microbial contaminations before use. Manufacturers can try to mitigate potential supply shortages in the future by contracting multiple suppliers. The trade off of having multiple suppliers is the average price for materials will be higher but still less expensive than dealing with a supply shortage in the future. Working with local suppliers is yet another way manufacturers attempt to reduce their variable costs of production.

Manufacturers also have indirect costs in the form of overhead. These costs are necessary for the manufacturer to function but are not directly related to a specific product. Examples of indirect costs are the IT systems, quality control systems, and management. These indirect costs can be high if the company only has a few products. Luckily, the overhead can be lowered if it can be spread across multiple products. Investing in systems that can streamline quality processes, will help reduce costs over the vaccine production lifetime for the company.

Regulatory, licensing, and commercialization costs are the last type of mixed costs that vaccine manufacturers face. Regulatory and licensing requirements are well documented by National Regulatory Authorities (NRAs). The requirements are relatively similar across each NRAs, but they can change due to significant events in the industry. These events may require the existing regulations to evolve or changes to be made in the enforcement of the regulatory measures. NRAs may have different licensing and compliance regulations which would mean certain lots of vaccines would need to be made specifically for certain countries. Manufacturers will need to pay the fees required to comply with the regulatory requirements as well as pay for the licenses to allow them to export their vaccines to other countries. Some countries that are receiving vaccines require country specific clinical trials.

The company will also be subject to routine NRA inspections. For large vaccine manufacturers, exporting to several countries, they will need to manage a large number of export licenses for each market their product is licensed in and be ready to have their facilities continually inspected by multiple NRAs. Beyond the licensing process, manufacturers also have the option to sell their product through other channels such as the United Nations Children's Emergency Fund (UNICEF) Supply Division, the Pan American Health Organization (PAHO), and other procurement organizations. These organizations may procure hundreds of millions of doses for their constituents, but manufacturers must first comply with the WHO Pre-Qualification (PQ) requirements. For some companies, additional processes will need to be developed and implemented in order to meet the PQ requirements. WHO also charges fees for vaccine PQ to provide financial stability to the program. Finally, commercialization costs refer to all expenses a company incurs to market and eventually sell their product. The total development costs to bring a vaccine to market can be roughly similar to that of pharmaceutical drugs (Institute of Medicine, 2003). Some experts estimate a new vaccine costs $700 million from initial research to commercial production. Modern vaccines are also subject to constant upgrades due to technological advances in production processes. For example the MMR vaccine currently being produced in the United States is far different from the version produced in 1971.

Patents
The continuous process of improving and modifying the manufacturing process can be a significant obstacle for companies as it can lead to delays and the need for additional testing to validate the new process (Plotkin et al., 2017). Therefore, companies place a lot of emphasis in creating an optimal manufacturing process as early into the development stage as possible (Plotkin et al., 2017). The immediate impact of removing suboptimal processes is that it enables manufacturing companies to be the first in the market with new biopharmaceuticals. History has shown

that being the first in the market is a major success factor for these companies. The life cycle of vaccines tends to be long and having an optimized manufacturing process will help generate cost savings over the entire vaccine life-cycle. However, companies also need to balance the need to be first to penetrate the market and risk not fully optimizing the manufacturing process. Regardless of which goal the manufacturing company decides to focus on, they will lock in their process and protect it from other companies by filing for a patent.

Patents are also used by manufacturers to protect property rights, which helps encourage companies to proceed with vaccine R&D (Institute of Medicine, 2003). The patent is awarded to the company that is able to establish proof they were the first to create a new product. The patent will prohibit non patent holders from marketing the product for 17 years. Without a patent, competitors would be free to reverse engineer the product without having the substantial R&D costs that the patent holder incurred during the development of the product. During this guaranteed market exclusivity, the patent holder can collect profits to start paying off all the R&D, production, and regulatory costs incurred up until that point. Furthermore, the patent holder will create a monopoly market and is free to charge monopoly prices. In general, the profits in a monopoly market is proportional to the market demand the price society is willing to pay for the vaccine. Understanding the market demand and societies willingness to pay plays a critical role in influencing vaccine manufacturers to decide which projects to pursue.

While the patent system is beneficial, it does come with some limitations. Patents raise prices and may lead to decreased outputs. This can occur, when some patients who would generally pay for competitively priced vaccines decide to not pay for vaccines priced under a monopoly system. Patents also raise an ethical dilemma. When a single manufacturer has the right to produce all the vaccines, there will often be a limit to how many vaccines are produced. As a result, wealthier countries will often be more successful in purchasing and securing vaccines for their citizens over low income countries (Brock, 2021). This raises the question if this divide in vaccine distribution is ethically acceptable.

Take the current COVID-19 pandemic for example, the global infection rate in India reached 314 000 with 4000 dying every day. Other countries such as Mexico and Brazil also face high infection rates but lack the medical resources to tackle the issue. In the United States, most of the citizens have been vaccinated and they are moving to vaccinate teenagers who have low risk of complications from COVID-19. But the countries with record high infection rates still have not received enough vaccines to fully vaccinate their health care workers, much less their vulnerable elderly population. Therefore, some argue that by waiving some rights of the vaccine patent will allow other countries to produce generic copies of the vaccine and increase the global supply of vaccines. This will give developing countries the much needed access to vaccines and help save lives and decrease the prevalence of future variants from appearing. Unfortunately, the patent is the only thing that protects the vaccine manufacturer and allows them to start covering their expenses that went into the production of the vaccine. Without the protection from patents, vaccine manufacturers would have no incentive to spend the money on R&D for future vaccines.

Revenue Structure

In 2013, the total vaccine sales for infectious diseases were more than $25 billion worldwide (3). Despite the anti-vaccines movement, the vaccine market continues to grow. According to a survey conducted by Zion Market Research, the total revenue from vaccines in 2014 was around $32.2 billion (Doughman, 2019). By 2020, the total global revenue is expected to reach $59.2 billion, almost double what was seen in 2014 (Doughman, 2019).

Large multinational manufacturers sell vaccines through a two-tiered pricing system (Institute of Medicine, 2003). The first tier is to sell vaccines to developed countries at a high price. The second tier is to sell vaccines at a low price, often at or close to the manufacturer's marginal costs, to developing countries. The first tier accounts for 82 percent of the vaccine revenue, but only accounts for around 12 percent of the total doses. The remaining 88 percent of the doses are distributed to the developing countries for minimal profit. However, this system works because it allows the vaccine manufacturers to exploit economies of scale when producing their large global volume of vaccines, which keeps their average costs low. The manufacturers are then able to sell their vaccines to developed countries and earn extremely high returns while simultaneously distributing much needed vaccines to developing countries and assisting them in their vaccination protocols. European multinational vaccine manufacturers will typically produce hundreds of millions of doses, while comparable United States multinational vaccine manufacturers will only produce ten of millions of doses (Institute of Medicine, 2003). Due to the disparity in the volume of vaccines produced between the United States and Europe, the United States faces higher average costs compared to Europe. Additionally the costs of producing vaccines have been generally increasing, while revenue from vaccine sales have remained generally constant. Unlike prescription drugs which can be taken for years by patients, vaccines are generally administered within one to four doses over the patient's lifetime. This greatly limits the total revenue vaccine manufacturers can expect to generate from each individual. Additional revenue pressures are applied when the CDC negotiates lower federal contract prices, which may include price caps for some vaccines. The constantly increasing number of vaccines purchased by governments at discounted prices and the price competition between different government contracts all have a negative impact on revenue.

Summary

The business side of vaccine production and distribution is a long and complex system. There are considerable risks that are taken on by vaccine manufacturers when deciding to spend money on the R&D for new vaccine development. The substantial initial investment required to enter the vaccine manufacturing industry serves as a significant barrier to entry. Vaccine manufacturers that are successful in creating a novel product are rewarded with the ability to sell their product as a monopoly to recoup their initial investments and secure profits. Patents play a large role in a companies ability to protect their novel property and production process from their competitors. Once the patent expires, the monopoly market will transition to a price taker market, where prices will generally be more stable.

Chapter 8: Benefits Of Inoculation And Prevention

Vaccination is an easy and safe way to prevent diseases and ultimately save lives. There are vaccines to protect against at least 20 different diseases around the world and together they have saved the lives of over 3 million people a year (World Health Organization [WHO], 2020). There are multiple benefits to getting vaccinated, including protecting yourself from potentially life threatening diseases, protecting the people around you, preventing the spread of variants, and helping eradicate diseases.

Herd Immunity
When a person gets a vaccine, they are training their body's natural immune system to recognize and fight a specific bacteria or virus. If the person is infected with the disease after vaccination, the body will be equipped with memory B-cells and memory T-cells that are ready to quickly destroy the invasive pathogen. In most cases, the invasive pathogen is destroyed before the host displays symptoms of the illness. The most direct effect of getting a vaccine is that an individual is protecting themselves from getting the disease. However, there is another indirect effect that can occur as more people start to get vaccinated. Vaccinated individuals have a reduced risk of transmitting a disease to others. In general, a disease does not have time to become transmittable in the body of a vaccinated individual, because of how quickly it is destroyed by the immune system. This significantly reduces

the likelihood a vaccinated person would be able to transmit a bacterial or viral infection to others. When the majority of the general population starts to become vaccinated, we can observe a protective effect known as herd immunity (Kim et al., 2011; WHO, 2020). This is an effect that is not observed in unvaccinated populations. Herd Immunity can be achieved when immunity to a specific disease is generated after natural infection or through a high proportion of vaccinated individuals in the population (Randolph & Barreiro, 2020; WHO, 2020). The first option is not extremely viable as a large fraction of the population would need to contract the disease and millions would succumb to it (Randolph & Barreiro, 2020). Therefore, policies are often implemented to help prevent the spread of the disease and reduce transmission rates until herd immunity is achieved through vaccinations.

Herd immunity is extremely helpful in society because some subpopulations may not be able to take vaccines. For example, immunocompromised individuals or extremely young children are generally not able to be vaccinated. Therefore, they rely on the general population and herd immunity to protect them. The way herd immunity works is that it prevents the spread of a contagious disease by having it destroyed by a vaccinated individual's immune system. If a vaccinated individual is exposed to a disease causing pathogen, their immune system will generally be able destroy the pathogen before they become symptomatic and start transmitting the disease to others. In the rare case the vaccinated individual transmits the disease, in a population with a high proportion of inoculated people, they will probably spread to other vaccinated people thus limiting the opportunity it has to spread. In general, the spread of the disease is stopped quickly and efficiently since vaccines are effective at stopping the transmission of illnesses from occurring. As a result, individuals that are not vaccinated have a very small risk of being exposed to a life threatening disease from a vaccinated person.

The importance of herd immunity was first recognized when combating smallpox (Kim et al., 2011). The goal was to have 80% of the population inoculated in order to achieve the herd immunity effect. The mass vaccination programmes were successful in significantly reducing the number of small cases in endemic countries. There are many examples of vaccination programmes that are currently in place that use herd immunity to help protect people and prevent the spread of diseases.

Vaccination against the invasive Haemophilus influenza type b with the conjugate vaccine resulted in a decline in disease prevalence in vaccinated populations (Kim et al., 2011). The herd immunity effect was seen once 50% of the population was inoculated. Most importantly, after the introduction of the vaccine, there was a reduction of infections in unvaccinated older children over the age of 5. Herd immunity can also be seen in pertussis-related cases. Pertussis is a disease that can give rise to severe complications such as pneumonia, seizures, subdural bleeding, and hernias or result in death (Government of Canada, 2018). The majority of mortalities from pertussis occur in infants less than three months old. However, the routine immunization schedule for infants recommends infants receive the first dose of the vaccine at 2 months (Government of Canada, 2018). Therefore, it is better to protect infants through the use of herd immunity (Kim et al., 2011). Adults are given a booster pertussis vaccination to maintain vaccine efficacy in the population. Other examples such as measles, mumps, polio and chickenpox, are all infectious diseases that are now rare since we established herd immunity through vaccinations (Rogers & Health, 2021). In 2019, we saw a measles outbreak originating from Disneyland (Krakow, 2019). These outbreaks can occur because the vaccine coverage in the areas are low and does not provide herd immunity protection to the population (Rogers & Health, 2021). WHO supports reaching herd immunity through vaccinations, because it prevents the spread of a disease through a population which would result in unnecessary deaths (WHO, 2020). A complication of herd immunity is that some diseases do not have vaccines. Even if a lot of adults have developed immunity to these diseases because of prior infection, the disease can still circulate through the children and infect others with weakened immune systems (Rogers & Health, 2021). Additionally, herd immunity is limited to protecting against diseases that are spread person-to-person (WHO, 2020). Diseases such as tetanus, which is contracted from a bacteria in the environment and not from other people, would not benefit from herd immunity. Unimmunized persons would still contract the disease even if the majority of the population were vaccinated.

COVID-19

In order to reach herd immunity against the SARS-CoV-2 virus which causes COVID-19, experts suggest we need at least 70% of the population to be inoculated to achieve herd immunity (Rogers & Health, 2021). If the SARS-CoV-2 virus is like other coronaviruses that currently infect humans, we can expect that people who get infected and fight off the illness will remain immune for months to years. This hypothesis has been confirmed in population-based studies conducted in Denmark, which showed that people who have been previously infected by SARS-CoV-2 virus are protected against repeated infection for more than six months. While this is positive news for the healthy population, the same level of immunity is unlikely to be seen in immunocompromised individuals or the older generation with weaker immune systems.

To further complicate the issue, COVID-19 virus is prone to mutations called variants. This is normal with all viruses, and in most cases, mutations are useless and go undetected (Ries, 2021)., Every time the virus infects a new host it has a chance to mutate and due to number of people getting infected by COVID-19 globally, some health experts are concerned a new variant may decrease the effectiveness of the vaccination programmes currently in place (Rogers & Health, 2021). Variants can increase transmission rates and make the disease outbreak harder to control, which will only prolong the pandemic. The first variant, D614G, appeared in Australia and India in May (Ries, 2021). Followed by the B.1.1.7 variant in the United Kingdom and the B.1.351 variant in South Africa. More variants have now been discovered in Los Angeles and Ohio. The B.1.1.7 variant is thought to be 50% more contagious than previous variants and the CDC expects it to be the dominant strain in the United States. The B.1.351 variant has a mutation in the spike protein where it binds to human cells. This increases the survivability of the virus in vaccinated individuals. In fact, Moderna is working on a vaccine booster shot to target this variant and Pfizer stated that their current vaccine will be slightly less effective on this variant.

Despite having multiple effective vaccines currently being

administered globally, it is difficult to predict the future and know when we will have achieved herd immunity. Some experts predict that it may no longer be possible to eradicate COVID-19 due to all the variants around the world. As mentioned previously, a study in Denmark found that infected individuals had immunity to reinfection for over six months (Rogers & Health, 2021). Other studies have results that indicate that the antibodies created to fight the virus decreased over time and in some cases was not sufficient to prevent reinfection (Anderson et al., 2020; Randolph & Barreiro, 2020). While more studies will need to be conducted to assess the duration of long term immunity to the SARS-CoV-2 virus, most studies are indicating that human's immunity to the coronavirus decreases over time. This indicates that we would not be able to achieve persistent herd immunity and instead require to update the vaccine and provide booster doses through a routine vaccination programme.

Eradication of Disease
Vaccinations have had an enormous contribution to global health (Greenwood, 2014). Since the creation of WHO's Expanded Programme of Immunization in 1974 and the Global Alliance for Vaccination and Immunization in 2000, the global vaccination coverage of many infectious diseases have been drastically improved. Other initiatives such as One Health, endorsed by the CDC, focus on tackling disease prevention, treatment, and eradication (Corona, 2020). Successfully eradicating a disease is the ultimate goal for health officials, as it results in better health and benefits the ecosystems on a global level. Eradication of a disease is defined as "permanent reduction to zero of the worldwide incidence of infection caused by a specific agent as a result

of deliberate efforts" and is widely accepted by many organizations including the WHO (Corona, 2020).

To date, WHO has declared two major infectious diseases to be officially eradicated: smallpox and rinderpest (Corona, 2020; Greenwood, 2014). Smallpox was a deadly disease that caused epidemics throughout human history and resulted in 300 - 500 million deaths in the 20th century (Corona, 2020). The smallpox vaccine was the first vaccine to be widely distributed and fittingly smallpox was the first disease to be eradicated through vaccinations (Greenwood, 2014). The last case of smallpox was reported in Somalia in 1977 and was declared as eradicated in 1980. Smallpox is also the only human infection to have been eradicated. Rinderpest was a bovine disease, closely related to measles and distemper viruses, that caused the death of cattle herds throughout Europe and Africa from the 18th to the 20th century (Corona, 2020; Greenwood, 2014). The disease would wipe out herds of cattle in developing countries, resulting the many families losing their food source and becoming malnourished and susceptible to other infectious diseases (Greenwood, 2014). The last reported case of rinderpest occurred in Kenya in 2001 and was officially declared as eradicated in 2011.

Attempts to eradicate other diseases are proving to be more difficult. Both smallpox and rinderpest had characteristics that helped facilitate their eradication. Based on the scientific data and the their respective eradication campaigns, health officials and scientists have created a checklist to determine if a disease can be eradicated (Corona, 2020):

- Is the disease easily diagnosable or recognizable?
- Is there a non-human reservoir or vector (or both)?

- Is the disease geographically restricted?
- Is there a vaccine? Are there other transmission-disrupting alternatives?

Is the disease easily diagnosable or recognizable?
The symptoms of a disease is one the ways to quickly diagnose the presence of a disease in an individual or community. In the case of smallpox, the characteristic sores and rashes allowed health officials to diagnose outbreaks easily and effectively in their communities. In general, the more complicated the method to diagnose a disease, the less likely it will be eradicated. This is evident in the case of malaria. Historically, professionals were required to interpret the patient's blood smears in order to identify infected individuals. The lack of trained professionals in endemic areas led to the eventual failure of the campaign to eradicate malaria.

Is there a non-human reservoir or vector (or both)?
It is not uncommon for disease to be able to infect multiple organisms. For example, SARS, caused by SARS-CoV, can infect humans despite not being the original host for this virus. It is believed that the non-human reservoir for the SARS-CoV is in bats. Despite SARS transmissions between people being successfully stopped, the existence of a non-human reservoir allows for a chance for reinfection in the future. In some cases, pathogens have adapted to using one organism as a host to help transmit to another host species. For example, dengue fever is transmitted to people through mosquito vectors.

Mosquitos are hosts that carry the pathogen, while displaying little to no symptoms of the disease. Similar to SARS, even if the disease was eliminated from the human population, the existence of a non-human reservoir can allow for reinfection in the future. Since the smallpox virus only infected humans, it was able to be eradicated through targeted vaccination campaigns. Like smallpox, the poliovirus only infect humans and have been eliminated in 193 countries and are close to being fully eradicated.

Yellow fever is an example of a disease that saw its incidence drop to zero due to vaccination efforts in Nigeria. However, yellow fever virus has non-human reservoirs and in conjunction with decreasing vaccination rates, there was an outbreak of yellow fever in 2017. Now Nigeria experiences seasonal yellow fever outbreaks.

Is the disease geographically restricted?
Many diseases that are being targeted for eradication by the WHO, such as polio, malaria, measles, and rubella, can be observed in multiple countries. However, as a disease approaches eradication, it tends to become more geographically restricted. This has a couple of effects. The nations that have zero disease incidence may start to scale back their eradication campaigns since they see no changes in societal, political, and economical benefits by continuing on. However, this is a problem as the regions that still have disease incidences may still require support from other nations. This is a problem that is currently being observed in the polio eradication campaign. The benefit of a restricted geographical region is that the eradication campaigns can focus on targeting areas where it is most needed instead of global mass coverage. Some diseases such as guinea worm disease have never spread globally and as a result have been able to be pushed to the brink of eradication with targeted

campaigns.

Is there a vaccine? Are there other transmission-disrupting alternatives?

Vaccines were responsible for the eradication of smallpox and rinderpest and are the foundation for the majority of the ongoing disease elimination campaigns. But some scientists question if eradication of disease can only occur through the use of vaccines. The disease dracunculiasis, or guinea worm disease, is caused through the ingestion of Dracunculus medinensis larvae from contaminated water sources. Currently there are no therapeutics or vaccines to treat dracunculiasis. However, guinea worm disease is close to eradication despite the lack of vaccines. Using different infectious disease containment strategies, the reduction in disease incidence was achieved using water filtration systems and potable drinking water. These systems and community education have helped reduce the number of cases from 3.5 million in 1986 to 53 cases in 2019. If guinea worm disease is completely eradicated, it will also be the first disease to be eradicated without the use of a vaccine. This would suggest that there are potentially multiple ways to eradicate diseases without having to rely on vaccines.

Smallpox and rinderpest were not just eradicated due to their scientific context. The eradication campaigns also required political, economic and social education efforts. Coordination and collaboration between nations is necessary to track outbreaks and mobilize resources efficiently. Political support is necessary for global health initiatives to work and social education programs are necessary to help tackle the global rise in mistrust in science, as evidenced by the rise of the anti-vaccination movement.

Moving Forward

Some organizations, including the WHO, are shifting towards using the term "disease elimination" instead of eradication due to its less stringent and more attainable definition (Corona, 2020). The disease elimination definition "does not require the permanent worldwide reduction of disease incidence to zero, but rather reducing incidence to zero in a particular geographic area" (Corona, 2020). This definition inspires more confidence in global health initiatives and an example can be seen in the declaration of cholera being eliminated from countries like Peru despite not being eradicated globally.

Currently there are multiple diseases on the brink of eradication including (Breene, 2017; Corona 2020):

- Poliovirus
- Dracunculiasis (guinea worm disease)
- Yaws
- Measles
- Mumps
- Rubella

The guinea worm virus is set to become the second human disease in history to be eradicated (Breene, 2017). The poliovirus has been successfully eliminated in 193 countries with outbreaks limited to Afghanistan, Nigeria, and Pakistan (Corona, 2020). Measles has been eliminated from most affluent countries due to vaccination programmes, but with the rise of the anti-vaccine movement and an increase in unvaccinated children, there has been a rise in localised measles outbreaks (Breene, 2017). Despite these setbacks, WHO hopes to eliminate the disease globally within the next couple of years. Mumps outbreaks are rare due to the "MMR vaccine" given to children. Rubella is a disease that has been successfully eliminated from the Americas, and its prevalence is being targeted and reduced in other nations.

The benefits of vaccination and prevention of diseases is the protection of human life. Vaccinations prevent the spread of life threatening diseases and help protect nations from mass loss of life due to uncontrolled spread of these diseases. Vaccination campaigns and programmes all aim to help create herd immunity to limit the spread of diseases and limit the opportunity for the disease to mutate into a variant. In the end, the eradication of a highly infectious disease helps protect our overall global health and ecosystem.

Chapter 9: Events That Left Trauma

Although the existence of vaccines has done much good for the citizens of the world by treating diseases and eradicating some, such as polio and smallpox, there is still skepticism held towards what motivation there is behind the development of a vaccine. The methodology behind the testing of vaccines when the first vaccines were being distributed consisted of many questionable tactics, as well as an unethical use of test subjects, thus raising the question by many of how vaccines today are being tested and who or what the test subjects are. Also, many people do not understand how vaccines are developed, and the lengthy process that is required for a vaccine to enter a clinical trial before applying for approval.

Therefore, there is a great fear of the minor risks that are still present when administering a vaccine. Even though all medication has some forms of side effects, there are people who come up with various conspiracy theories in order to drive people away from wanting to receive treatment. In addition, certain historical events allow particular groups of people to hold negative views towards receiving vaccinations due to the generational trauma incurred by the past ulterior motives for administering vaccines. Vaccines used to serve a different agenda than treating and eradicating disease, and have left a large impact on those who have been given the vaccine, as well as on their families. This chapter will cover how traumatic historical events influence today's decisions, as well as how people choose to be bearers of fear, thus negatively impacting the points of view of those around them.

An Issue of Ethics

The invention of vaccines is a large reason for public health successes around the globe, however, vaccines are also a subject of several controversies that surround the issue of ethics (The History of Vaccines, 2018). Many ethical debates when it comes to vaccines and how they are regulated, developed, and used are related to the various components such as policies placed by the government, the nature of the research and testing of vaccines, how citizens are being informed of the vaccines they receive, and whether the vaccine is available to everyone (The History of Vaccines).

Vaccine Mandates

When the government places policies that state vaccine mandates, citizens are then required to receive vaccination. These mandates have also been incorporated into the school setting, where students must receive vaccination in order to be granted entry to their school. The first requirement for students to receive vaccination before being given permission to attend school was constituted in the 1850s for smallpox prevention (The History of Vaccines). Similar efforts were also enacted in the 1960s and 1970s in an effort to eradicate measles in the United States of America. Certain immunizations then became a requirement across the country by the 1990s (The History of Vaccines). These mandates are conceived based on the results that were obtained from the vaccine's clinical trials, as well as its performance upon being monitored further after being licensed.

Although the purpose of vaccine mandates is to attempt to

eradicate the disease(s) being combatted, there are several objections that need to be taken into consideration. The mandates may strive to protect the welfare of society, there are many groups within said society that may feel their interests are not being taken into account, as the regulations conflict with their religious and/or philosophical beliefs. Therefore, these public health vaccine regulations fall at risk of causing strain between the people and the government as "medical and public health advocates often struggle to balance the ethics of protecting individual beliefs and the community's health" (The History of Vaccines, 2018, para. 5).

The Research and Testing of Vaccines

In order to be licensed, several years worth of research is conducted, and the vaccine "must pass rigorous safety and efficacy standards" (The History of Vaccines, 2018, para. 7). A diverse group of experts is required for the vaccine research and development process from different fields "including public health, epidemiology, immunology, and statistics, and from pharmaceutical companies" (The History of Vaccines, 2018, para. 7). These different backgrounds imply there are different goals and/or methods between disciplines. This thus leads to "conflicting priorities and motives, which contributes to various ethical discussions" (The History of Vaccines, 2018, para. 7).

When a vaccine is being tested, test subjects are required in order to see how the treatment will interact with the immune system it enters. However, before humans are allowed to be test subjects, animals with similar DNA to humans are used to test the efficacy of the vaccine being tested. This is to ensure that any humans who sign up to be test subjects during the vaccine's clinical trials are not being exposed to potentially harmful substances in the vaccine. However, further precautions must be taken, hence why researchers disagree at times when it comes to who should be included in vaccine trials. For example, when testing certain vaccines, those with certain medical conditions cannot participate in the clinical trials because they fall at a higher risk of experiencing severe side effects. Therefore, in order to "properly test a vaccine's effectiveness, a clinical trial including a control group that does not get the test vaccine is usually necessary. Failing to provide any adequate preventive option can be a difficult decision when the vaccine can potentially prevent a serious, untreatable, or fatal infection" (The History of Vaccines, 2018, para. 8). Vaccines such as the Bacillus Calmette-Guérin (BCG) , that was used to treat tuberculosis, are not completely effective, and therefore can be extremely detrimental to those with damaged immune systems (The History of Vaccines).

Not only is it crucial to consider a vaccine's interactions with immune systems of varying strengths, but also how safe and effective it is in certain demographics. For example, when a vaccine is being developed, researchers need to find a way to safely administer the vaccine to children as well. Therefore, several questions of ethics are posed as "researchers must balance the need to protect children's safety with the need to adequately understand how a vaccine will perform and protect children when administered" (The History of Vaccines, 2018, para. 9). It is additionally important to consider how the research, development, and distribution of a vaccine can affect those who are living in developing countries. Vaccine research that is hosted in developing countries raise many concerns as researchers need to determine what aspects of their research and/or development are necessary, such as treatment that will be administered if any diseases are detected (The History of Vaccines). Also, researchers must "ensure the trial and vaccine can be supervised by local ethical review panels", and "that participants understand consent" (The History of Vaccines, 2018, para. 10). Making sure that communication has been effective throughout the research, development, and distribution processes allows research participants and patients to be aware of any risks, such as side effects, and the actions they are entitled to take, such as withdrawing for any reason from the vaccine research study, or from receiving it.

Researchers also enter debates of ethics that discuss informed consent during the delivery of a vaccine. Patients who are about to receive a vaccine should be informed of the type of treatment that will be administered to them, as well as any potential risks they will be taking when receiving treatment. Although those who oppose this believe requiring consent will elicit unnecessary fear in patients, providing them with informed consent allows them to possess proper comprehension of the procedure, as well as leaves them room to ask questions and/or opt out of the treatment if they end up feeling uncomfortable. Therefore, it is specified in federal guidelines for healthcare providers to communicate with their patients. Even though it is not a necessity to "require written consent before vaccination (as they do for certain other procedures, such as surgeries), the National Childhood Vaccine Injury Act of 1986 requires that doctors give vaccine recipients, or their parents or legal representatives, a Vaccine Information Statement (VIS). The VIS provides basic information about vaccine risks and benefits and is designed to provide the information a patient or parent needs to make an informed decision" (The History of Vaccines, 2018, para. 12).

Concerns with Accessing Vaccines

Another ethical debate related to vaccines is whether the vaccine(s) will be distributed to everyone regardless of their socioeconomic status and/or their status as a member of a marginalized group, such as a minority race or ethnicity. Vaccines are predominantly provided by nations who are further developed and at a better financial standing compared to other countries, therefore, "implicit in these discussions is the question of whether or not all lives are of equal value, and equally deserving of opportunities to be protected by vaccination" (The History of Vaccines, 2018, para. 14).

The research and development of vaccines can be greatly inhibited by various aspects, such as the accountability researchers have to take due to the risks that accompany their test study, how much time and money the research requires, and when demand for the vaccine being tested is not as high anymore (The History of Vaccines). Most healthcare providers and world leaders inherently want what is best for their country and its people, therefore the decisions they make are influenced by the fact they prioritize their own nations' welfare over others. To experts who wish to make a considerably positive impact on public health, it would be a more ethical decision to increase the number of members in the vaccine production team. However, "when vaccines are in short supply, medical providers must make decisions about who should be protected, and who must be left vulnerable to disease" (The History of Vaccines, 2018, para. 15). Thus, when developing countries deal with public health crises that are not well known in developed nations, there is a lag in vaccine development as the developing countries do not possess the proper facilities to support wide-spread vaccine development and administering, while the developed nations do not familiarize themselves with the infections as they prioritize their own community health needs. These decisions therefore lead to supreme global health disparities.

Generational Trauma- Studying Sexually Transmitted Diseases

What is syphilis?
Syphilis is a bacterial infection that is also considered to be a sexually transmitted disease. This infection starts off as a sore on either the mouth, genitals, or rectum, and can spread from person to person when contact has been made with the sore, usually during sexual intercourse ("Syphilis-Symptoms and causes", 2018).

Syphilis can occur in multiple stages. The signs and symptoms change depending on the stage and its severity:

Primary syphilis: The first stage of syphilis is known as primary syphilis. This is the least severe occurrence of syphilis, the infection starting out with a "firm, round, and painless" sore (CDC, 2019, para. 3). These sores are called chancres, and can be found anywhere around the mouth, genitals, anus or in the rectum, and can usually heal within three to six weeks. When bacteria has entered the body, a single chancre or several chancres can form in that area. Due to the fact that the chancres are typically painless, most people who have syphilis will not notice them, especially if the sores are located in the vaginal or rectum areas, making them more difficult to notice.

Secondary syphilis: The next stage of syphilis is called secondary syphilis. Similarly to primary syphilis, the signs and symptoms of this stage are mild and therefore can go unnoticed by those infected (CDC, 2019). In this stage, a non-irritating rash starting at the posterior and ultimately spreading throughout the whole body will develop within a few weeks of the chancre from the healing from the previous stage. Sores that appear to look like warts will also form in the mouth and genital area. In some cases, there are also occurrences of "hair loss, muscle aches, a fever, a sore throat and swollen lymph nodes" ("Syphilis-Symptoms and causes", 2018, para. 6). The signs and symptoms in secondary syphilis can either disappear in the span of a few weeks or inconsistently persist for up to a year.

Latent syphilis: The third stage of syphilis is called latent syphilis, where there are no signs or symptoms to be experienced. This stage can last for several years.

Tertiary syphilis: The last stage of syphilis is referred to as tertiary syphilis, a stage that "about 15% to 30% of people infected with syphilis who don't get treatment will develop" ("Syphilis-Symptoms and causes", 2018, para. 8). This stage is the most dangerous stage as it is "associated with severe medical problems" (CDC, 2019, para. 3). Many years after the initial infection, late stage syphilis can greatly damage several organs and other parts of the body such as the "brain, nerves, eyes, heart, blood vessels, liver, bones and joints" ("Syphilis-Symptoms and causes", 2018, para. 8).

How did syphilis start?
Although the exact origin of the disease still has not been determined, two hypotheses have been agreed upon: first, that the sailors who were with Christopher Columbus on his expedition to India brought the disease with them back

to Europe ("The History of Syphilis", 2017). The second hypothesis is that the disease was already existing in Europe and was viewed as leprosy ("The History of Syphilis").

The first outbreak of syphilis that was recorded in Europe occurred in Naples, Italy in 1495 ("The History of Syphilis", 2017). The reason it was viewed as leprosy at the time was because the symptoms would transform from "genital ulcers [that] led to fevers, rash, and joint and muscle pains" to "sores [that ate] into the bones and destroy various parts of the body including the nose, lips and eyes" ("The History of Syphilis", 2017, para. 3). Due to the lack of resources and understanding of this newly realized disease, most cases of syphilis led to the death of several people within the population. "Scandinavian countries [Norway, Sweden, Denmark, Finland, and Iceland], Britain, Hungary, Greece, Poland and Russia" began to deal with cases of syphilis by the 1500s, many of these countries blaming each other for the start of the disease due to their pre-existing rivalries ("The History of Vaccines", 2017, para. 4). Eventually, during those years (the sixteenth century), less fatalities were being recorded as syphilis was becoming less calamitous.

How was syphilis treated?
In the 1500s, guaiacum, a tree commonly found in the Caribbean area as well as tropical America, and topical ointments of mercury, a highly toxic metallic element, were used as treatments for syphilis before it was realized that mercury brought further damage to the body rather than act as a healing agent against the disease. Salvarsan, a drug that consists of antimicrobials (agents that either inhibit the growth of microorganisms or kill them) was used to treat syphilis in the early twentieth century. Soon after,

other treatments for the disease were discovered, such as Neosalvarsan and penicillin. Once penicillin started being used, the previously discovered and used "were found obsolete and syphilis was able to [be] effectively treated" ("The History of Vaccines", 2017, para. 7). Nowadays, along with penicillin, tetracycline and doxycycline- all antibiotics- are used to treat syphilis.

Syphilis Vaccine Development
Due to how widespread the syphilis disease became over time, as well as several public health efforts not going as planned, society's need to have access to an effective syphilis vaccine became more prominent.

Researchers had confidence in the syphilis vaccine being a success due to the fact that:

> *"(1) research community's accumulated knowledge of immune correlates of protection; (2) existence of a relevant animal model that enables effective preclinical analyses; (3) universal penicillin susceptibility of T. pallidum which enhances the attractiveness of clinical vaccine trials; and (4) significant public health benefit a vaccine would have on reduction of infectious/ congenital syphilis and HIV rates" (Cameron & Lukehart, 2014, para. 1).*

Currently, there is no vaccine effective enough to aid in the prevention of syphilis. Treponema pallidum, a spirochaete, has proven to be quite difficult to study due to its fragility and how it falls apart at minimal amounts of manipulation or how it does not grow in a laboratory setting due to it being "temperamental" (McRae, 2018, para. 6). Therefore, no vaccines were able to be developed for people to be immune to syphilis (McRae).

The Tuskegee Syphilis Study

The Tuskegee Syphilis Study, officially named the "Tuskegee Study of Untreated Syphilis in the Negro Male" was a research study at the Tuskegee Institute in Macon County, Alabama (The Editors of Encyclopaedia Britannica, 2019, para. 1). Originally scheduled to last for six to nine months, the Tuskegee Syphilis Study went on for forty years from 1932 to 1972. This study was coordinated by the U.S. Public Health Service in order to examine the development of syphilis in African American men: "whether syphilis caused cardiovascular damage more often than neurological damage and to determine if the natural course of syphilis in black men was significantly different from that in whites" (The Editor of Encyclopaedia Britannica, 2019, para. 2). Upon receiving the support of the Tuskegee Institute, a total of six hundred patients, most of whom were destitute sharecroppers, were enrolled in the research study with the promise of being provided with free healthcare. Three hundred and ninety-nine of them were infected with syphilis while the other two hundred and one were control patients as they were not infected with the disease. When they were recruited to participate in the study, all of the men were told that they were receiving treatment for "bad blood", which is a vague term as it describes a variety of illnesses. None of the six hundred research participants were told they had syphilis or the ways the disease can be transmitted from person to person, including through having sexual intercourse.

Although the initial plan of this research study was to make treatment a part of it as told to the research participants, "arsenic, bismuth, and mercury", all heavily toxic elements, were administered to the patients (The Editors of Encyclopedia Britannica, 2019, para. 3). Also, while being monitored by the health workers, the research participants were provided with "placebos such as aspirin and mineral supplements, despite the fact that penicillin became the recommended treatment for syphilis in 1947, some 15 years into the study" (Nix, 2019, para. 3). This is "in direct violation of government legislation that mandated the treatment of venereal disease" (The Editors of Encyclopedia Britannica, 2019, para. 3). When no data was obtained from the study, the U.S. Public Health Service decided to allow the disease to progress to the highest stage possible, thus putting a stop to all forms of treatment in the study and monitoring the test subjects until their deaths. Therefore, no help was provided to the test subjects as they "died, went blind or insane or experienced other severe health problems due to their untreated syphilis" (Nix, 2019, para. 4). This ultimately led to the death of more than one hundred of the test subjects whose conditions were left to progress to tertiary syphilis, the most dangerous and lethal stage of syphilis.

Peter Buxton, who was working in San Francisco as a Public Health Service venereal disease investigator, made his supervisors aware of the unethical Tuskegee Syphilis Study upon finding out about it in the mid-1960s. Despite the fact that a committee was formed to further investigate the study, it was ultimately decided to continue on with it, still with the goal of monitoring the test subjects until they have passed away (Nix). The story of the Tuskegee of Untreated Syphilis in the Negro Male made its way to the Associated Press's Jean Heller- writer and investigative journalist- who broke the story of the study in July 1972, eventually leaving the

Tuskegee Syphilis Study with no other option than to shut down. By the time the story was released, only seventy four people who were the original test subjects survived, "at least 40 spouses had been diagnosed with it and the disease had been passed to 19 children at birth" (Nix, 2019, para. 7).

Due to the unethical decisions made throughout the period of the Tuskegee Syphilis Study, not only did several uninformed research participants greatly suffer and die, their families were also heavily affected by the disease as well as the loss of their family members. As one of the main questions of this research study was on the basis of race, many still question today whether the Tuskegee Syphilis Study was an attempted genocide disguised as helpful scientific research. Some factors that further the suspicions of many citizens are that the study ended up lasting four decades instead of the originally planned six to nine months (approximately a 5233-7900% difference), despite the fact that it was difficult to obtain data during the study, thus leaving the researchers to decide to monitor the test subjects until their death, regardless of their evident suffering in the process. Therefore, over the years, "many African Americans developed a lingering deep mistrust of public health officials and vaccines" due to a great fear that history will repeat itself (Nix, 2019, para. 9).

The Guatemala Syphilis Experiment
The Guatemala Syphilis Experiment was an American medical research study that took place in Guatemala from 1946 to 1948. John C. Cutler, a United States Public Health Service scientist directed this study and had also conducted the Terre Haute Study and was also involved in the Tuskegee Syphilis Study. He and his team collaborated with local Guatemalan physicians and were thus provided access to "public health

centres, government hospitals, mental institutions, and orphanages" (Rogers, 2019, para. 4). This study was designed to test how effective several medications were when treating sexually transmitted diseases, such as syphilis. Some of these medications include penicillin, an antibiotic, and orvus-mapharsen, an aresnical agent. The Guatemala Syphilis Experiment is mainly known for the unethical approaches when conducting the study and its targeting of particularly vulnerable populations, which "included more than 5,500 Guatemalan prisoners, sex workers, soldiers, children, and psychiatric patients, about one-quarter of whom were deliberately infected with syphilis, gonorrhea, or chancroid and all of whom were enrolled in the experiments without their consent" (Rogers, 2019, para. 1).

Near the beginning of the Second World War, there was an issue with the soldiers from the United States military contracting sexually transmitted diseases due to their physical relationships with prostitutes. United States medical researchers were attempting to figure out an effective strategy to prevent these diseases, so when it was realized that penicillin could be a fast acting treatment against syphilis, the United States military started to use penicillin upon exposure to or contraction of sexually transmitted diseases. However, the Guatemala Syphilis Study was put forward due to the uncertainty of penicillin working effectively in the long-run when providing preventative protection against sexually transmitted diseases.

The study design of this experiment was very unethical due to the use of "normal exposure", where infected sex workers told to participate in the study were also told to sleep with unknowing prisoners in order to transmit the disease to them. This was in order to figure out immunization methods for gonorrhea, syphilis, and chancroid. The Guatemala Syphilis Study was conducted in a hospital that was built for the study and located in Guatemala City. The hospital had three hundred beds, thus having enough space to be able to house a large population of prisoners and other test subjects who will be participating in this experiment.

Around five thousand, five hundred people have participated in the Guatemala Syphilis Study, and approximately one thousand, three hundred and eight of them were deliberately administered sexually transmitted diseases throughout the duration of the study. Those infected consisted of "soldiers, prisoners, sex workers, and psychiatric patients, ranging from age 10 to 72" and were exposed to syphilis "through inoculation of the cervix in sex workers; through infection or direct sexual contact with infected sex workers in prisoners and through injection, inoculation (via abrasion) of the penis, cisternal puncture (the insertion of a needle below the occipital bone at the back of the skull to access cerebrospinal fluid), or oral ingestion in psychiatric patients". Those who were exposed to gonorrhea were done so via sex workers "through cervical inoculation and in Guatemalan soldiers through sexual contact with the sex workers and sometimes through urethral inoculation; psychiatric patients were infected through inoculation of the urethra, rectum, or eyes". Finally, Guatemalan soldiers and psychiatric patients contracted chancroid through "abrasion and rubbing of inoculum into the skin on the arms or back" (Rogers, 2019, para. 5). Dr. Cutler proceeded to start an STD treatment program in order to spread the word about his prophylaxis study as well as to make peace with the government of Guatemala. Eight hundred and twenty of the test subjects received treatment for their infections, though more than six hundred and fifty of those test subjects were placed in the deliberate exposure group.

A phase in this research study that lasted until 1953 with the objective to "refine diagnostic techniques for STD" included:

> "Serology testing, in which blood and spinal fluid samples were collected for the detection of antibodies and microorganisms indicative of infection, was performed in 5,128 subjects (some of whom were involved in the intentional infection arm of the study). Subjects included children as young as one year, persons with leprosy, psychiatric patients, and personnel stationed at the U.S. Air Force base in Guatemala. This phase of the research, intended to refine diagnostic techniques for STDs, lasted until 1953." (Rogers, 2019, para. 6).

After the Presidential Commission for the study of Bioethical Issues conducted a thorough investigation of Dr. John Cutler's colleagues did not agree with his methods, and that the test subjects were not compliant as they did not provide consent to take part in the experiment. He withheld information regarding his experiment from the Pan American Sanitary Bureau (PASB) due to his concerns that people who find out about his methods will disagree, thus putting his research study in jeopardy of being shut down.

The Terre Haute Prison Experiments
The design of the Guatemala Syphilis Experiment was also inspired by the Terre Haute prison experiments from 1943-1944 that took place in Guatemala and conducted by

researchers from Terre Haute, Indiana. Dr. John C. Cutler, a doctor two years out of medical school who also worked on the Tuskegee Syphilis Study experiments, was funded by the U.S. National Institutes of Health to conduct a study in Guatemala. He started his research in Terre Haute where he had obtained consent from prisoners taking part in the experiment to be infected with gonorrhea that had been contracted by prostitutes. However, he had difficulty with obtaining data for his study because he was not able to find a way to infect the men in a reliable manner, therefore he moved his study to Guatemala, where prostituion was legal. Thus, Dr. John C. Cutler was able to run his experiments through the use of a natural route of infection. Most of the test subjects who were participating in this part of Cutler's study were not told that they would be infected with different sexually transmitted diseases, thus leading Dr. John C. Cutler and his team to deliberately expose one thousand, three hundred people to these diseases.

The following are some more specific events that occurred during Dr. Cutler's experiments:

- "Prostitutes who tested positive for gonorrhea or syphilis could visit prisoners at Guatemala City's Central Penitentiary—all paid for by U.S. taxpayers," notes Wellesley professor Reverby in her paper on the experiments. She goes on to write, "the researchers actually timed how long they spent with the prostitutes and thought they acted 'like rabbits'." In a similar experiment with Guatemalan soldiers, records show a prostitute servicing 8 soldiers in 71 minutes.

- At National Psychiatric Hospital of Guatemala, the team

tried to infect asylum patients by scratching the arms, faces, or mouths of women and the penises of men with a needle full of syphilis bacteria. Hundreds of psychiatric patients were thus exposed to syphilis.

- The single most horrific case may be that of Berta, who was infected with syphilis but not treated for 3 months. As Matthew Walter describes in Nature, 'Her health worsened, and within another three months Cutler reported that she seemed close to death. He re-infected Berta with syphilis, and inserted pus from someone with gonorrhoea into her eyes, urethra and rectum. Over several days, pus developed in Berta's eyes, she started bleeding from her urethra and then she died.'" (Zhang, 2015, para. 11-13)

Testing treatments to prevent syphilis has been rendered impossible due to the fact that Dr. John Cutler was unable to find a reliable or effective method of exposure for him to infect the test subjects with the disease. Dr. John C. Cutler died in 2003, and so did many of the people he had participate in his experiments. Now, three generations later, researchers are having difficulties with developing a vaccine that will be effective enough to treat syphilis.

The following chapter will cover more reasons why vaccine hesitancy is still prevalent. What sorts of conspiracy theories do people come up with to catalyze doubt and fear in society, and what role does social media play in vaccine hesitancy?

Chapter 10: Conspiracies, COVID-19, And Social Media

Distrust in governments and the global pharmaceutical industry is not a novel issue. People have long speculated upon and come up with conspiracies regarding supposed hidden agendas of the government or sinister, ulterior motives of big pharma. Some conspiracies are logical, and some have even turned out to be true - but many conspiracies are often baseless and built on false beliefs, posing a dangerous threat to public health through misinformation. As well, the age of social media has allowed these theories - no matter how outlandish they may be - to be amplified through the internet and given platforms that reach thousands of people. According to Islam et al. (2021), people may be compelled to spread and share vaccination misinformation and conspiracy theories if they are constantly exposed to social media and the anti-vaccination movement online.

In the current era of COVID-19, conspiracies are particularly harmful as they can dissuade people from getting immunized and prolong the duration of the pandemic. Indeed, high numbers of vaccine refusals and unvaccinated or undervaccinated individuals in certain areas have been linked to outbreaks of diseases that would have otherwise been preventable through vaccines (Stein, 2017). However, anti-vaccination sentiment has a history that extends far beyond the start of this pandemic. This chapter will explore some of the popular conspiracies related to vaccines and

COVID-19 and uncover how and why they came to gain so much traction, as well as examine the background behind conspiracy theories on social media.

Social Media, the Good and the Ugly

Social media is a revolutionary tool. Through it, critical information about public health can be accessed by nearly anyone with a smartphone. People can learn about health issues, prevention, share knowledge, and listen to scientific opinions. Between 50-80% of people look to the internet for health related information annually, and this number is only increasing (Stein, 2017). However, with this, also comes the opportunity for misinformation to spread. And indeed, misinformation is shared vastly all over the internet every single day. On Facebook, a page titled "The Truth About Cancer", has over one million followers. The page is extremely active, posting multiple times a day and peddling claims that vaccines can cause brain damage, autism, cancer, dementia, or Parkinson's disease and suggesting that people should instead look to natural remedies for their illnesses.

A 2013 study by the Centers for Disease Control and Prevention (CDC) confirmed that vaccines are not linked with autism, adding to a plethora of research which had previously determined the same (Centers for Disease Control and Prevention, n.d.). Other studies have also debunked links between vaccinations and neurological disorders or cancer as urban myths (Gasparini et al., 2015; MacArthur et al., 2008). In fact, early childhood vaccination has actually been associated with decreasing the risk of leukemia (MacArthur et al., 2008). Despite this scientific evidence, the owners of the "The Truth About Cancer" page often write that drug companies are only looking out for profit, and not the best interest of public health and thus vaccines and modern medicine should not be trusted. In one post, they recommend a combination of coconut oil and cannabis as a substitute for medical treatment to fight cancer. The post has over 2,000 likes and 1,400 shares. The dangers of suggesting such natural remedies over treatment from licensed medical doctors and vaccines are apparent. According to the Center for Countering Digital Hate (CCDH), people who depended on social media for COVID-19 related news were less likely to get vaccinated in comparison to people who used traditional media for COVID-19 related news (Jimenez, 2021).

Similar pages and groups exist across other social media platforms. On Instagram, the hashtag "antivax" contains over 100,000 posts. Although many of those posts are from people actually advocating for vaccination, it is also easy to find content containing anti-vaccination messaging. Some of the top photos under the hashtag are memes suggesting that those who do choose to get vaccinated are research guinea pigs and even claims that vaccines are the work of the devil. On Reddit, a subreddit titled "r/DebateVaccines" is an active community with nearly 6,000 members, many of whom hold anti-vaccination sentiment and commonly share conspiracies about vaccines. Much of the debate occurring on the subreddit also attempts to use scientific evidence and reason, but the presence of implausible conspiracy theories and misinformation cannot be ignored. Because of the COVID-19 pandemic, many of the conspiracies posted to the subreddit are related to the COVID-19 vaccines. There are posts and comments claiming that the COVID-19 vaccines cause infertility in women, or that they were created as a plot to reduce the population in order to combat climate change, and even that people belonging to the elite class, such as Bill Gates, will be using the vaccines to control the rest of humanity. Reddit and Instagram are not alone in hosting conspiracy content such as this. Similar content can also be found on Twitter, YouTube, 4Chan, and all over the internet. Later in this chapter, some of the most popular theories on the internet related to vaccines will be examined further. But first, it is important to understand why conspiracy theories are even created, and how they are able to attract attention and gain prevalence.

The Psychology Behind Conspiracies

According to Douglas et al. (2017), people may create conspiracy theories and choose them as explanations for events instead of non-conspiracy explanations when conspiracy theories offer satisfaction for their epistemic, existential, and social motives. An individual's epistemic motivation includes their desire to acquire an accurate understanding of a situation and obtain a sense of certainty. In other words, a need to know and to be right. Conspiracy theories can fulfill this desire by offering individuals "broad, internally consistent explanations that allow [them] to preserve beliefs in the face of uncertainty and contradiction" (Douglas et al., 2017, para 3). When presented with a situation where information is unavailable, inaccurate, or conflicting, individuals may choose to believe in a conspiracy theory in order to maintain a coherent epistemic understanding of the world. Situations that are difficult to understand, such as 9/11, can often invite the creation of conspiracies as people try to make sense of and understand what has happened. Existential motivation, on the other hand, includes a desire to feel secure in and in control of one's environment. This desire is fulfilled by conspiracy theories as they can offer individuals "the opportunity to reject official narratives and feel that they possess an alternative account" and the ability to feel safer using "cheater detection, in which dangerous and untrustworthy individuals are recognized and the threat they posed is reduced or neutralized" (Douglas et al., 2017, para 6). The popular conspiracy that the COVID-19 pandemic was intentional and preplanned is a good example of a theory that fulfills this motive. By portraying an accidental situation as something designed, individuals can escape the reality that the world is sometimes a dangerous place, where bad things can just happen.

Indeed, conspiracy theories often increase in prevalence during times of social crisis, where there is a high amount of fear and uncertainty throughout society (van Prooijen and Douglas, 2017). Lastly, conspiracy theories can offer fulfillment of social motivation which includes the desire to belong, fit in, and have a positive sense of oneself and one's group. By attributing negative outcomes to others instead of oneself or one's group, conspiracies can absolve oneself of blame for an unfavourable outcome or position (Douglas et al., 2017). Overall, by construing random events as malicious, orchestrated plans, conspiracy theorists can be able to feel a sense of understanding and control, escape uncertainty, fear, and anxiety, and portray others as evil while maintaining the morality and integrity of their own self or group.

Interestingly however, exposure to conspiracy theories has actually been shown to make people feel more uncertain, feel a loss of autonomy and control, and lead to feelings of alienation and social frustration (Douglas et al., 2017). However, belief in conspiracies may thrive despite this, not because they satisfy our psychological needs well and not because there is credible evidence for the conspiracy, but rather because in the unlikely event that a conspiracy turns out to be true, not having believed in it would have been detrimental. In other words, belief in the conspiracy may act as a safety net. As well, when conspiracy theorists encounter evidence that contradicts their conspiracy beliefs, it is often brushed aside as a result of the conspiracy (Lewandowsky et al., 2013). This means that conspiracy theorists can encounter scientific evidence that directly disproves their theory, only to decide that the evidence is an intentional attempt to mislead the public and push a certain agenda forward. This creates an unhealthy outlook of skepticism, mistrust, paranoia, and confirmation bias, where the conspiracy theorist will tend to only search for and believe in information that confirms their pre-existing beliefs and suspicions.

Infertility

One of the most common claims about the COVID-19 vaccines is that they cause infertility in women. The claim initially arose after the European Medicines Agency was petitioned by a German epidemiologist, Wolfgang Wodarg, to press pause on the approval of the Pfizer vaccine. Wodarg claimed that because syncytin-1 - a crucial protein component of placenta - and the SARS-CoV-2 spike protein were close in genetic proximity, the body could mistakenly attack syncytin-1 and render women infertile after receiving an anti-SARS-CoV-2 vaccine. The claim has spread through social media like wildfire, not because of its credibility, but because of the fear it induces in the heart of nearly any woman who comes across it. However, Wodarg's theory is false. The Food and Drug Administration (FDA) website states that there is no scientific evidence to support the claim. The protein created through the mRNA instructions of the Pfizer and Moderna vaccines is distinctive to SARS-CoV-2 and is not the same as any protein involved in the formation of placenta. The spike protein and syncytin-1 only share tiny portions of the same genetic code, not enough to make them identical and cause the immune system to mistakenly create antibodies against syncytin-1 after vaccination (Goodman, 2021). If the theory were true, women across the globe would have also noticed infertility effects after natural COVID-19 infection, as it also invokes an immune response against the SARS-CoV-2 spike protein (Goodman, 2021). As well, women from the clinical trials of COVID-19 vaccines have been successful in getting pregnant after receiving their vaccine (Campbell, 2021). According to FDA safety data, there was no difference in the number of pregnancies for women in the placebo group and women in the vaccine group for the Pfizer vaccine clinical trials. There were also no adverse events reported related to pregnancy. Despite this evidence, the theory continues to thrive on social media, contributing to vaccine hesitancy and misinformation.

Microchips, 5G, and Bill Gates

To most, the idea of vaccines containing microchips to track and control the population seems absurd, and perhaps even laughable. But according to a survey of 1,640 people by YouGov, it is suggested that approximately 28% of Americans believe that the initiative for global vaccination against COVID-19 is part of a plan created by Bill Gates to implant us all with microchip hardware. Part of this theory is that companies could use the microchips and the 5G network to collect biometric data and control people. The microchip rumor initially arose after Bill Gates talked about potential "digital certificates" in the future involving special invisible ink tattoos which could be used to keep track of testing, recovery, and vaccination history. However, neither Bill Gates nor The Gates Foundation have made any mention of a microchip, except to tell BBC that the conspiracy was false. Even the digital certificate concept never made it to human trials. Regardless, public figures such as Robert F. Kennedy Jr. have helped share and popularize the conspiracy through social media. Robert F. Kennedy Jr. was actually reprimanded by Instagram in February of 2021 for spreading debunked claims about COVID-19 and vaccines. On YouTube, Adam Fannin, a polemical Baptist pastor, posted a video titled "Bill Gates - Microchip Vaccine Implants to fight Coronavirus" which received over 2 million views and further helped to popularize this conspiracy. Donald Trump's former political advisor, Roger Stone, appeared on The Joe Piscopo Show and stated that "... [Bill Gates] and other globalists are definitely using [COVID-19] in a drive for mandatory vaccinations and microchipping people".

Despite their claims being baseless, fear mongering through social media allowed the theory to snowball and gain traction - even getting picked up by The New York Times. However, the theory has no footing. The COVID-19 vaccines are stored in clear vials, which contain six doses each. Implanting people with microchips from these vials simply would not be feasible. As well, the ingredients of every vaccine are available to the public, easily accessible through a Google search. For the Pfizer-BioNTech vaccine, the FDA lists the ingredients on their website: mRNA, lipids ((4-hydroxybutyl)azanediyl) bis(hexane-6,1-diyl)bis(2-hex-yldecanoate), 2 [(polyethylene glycol)-2000]-N,N-ditetradecylacetamide, 1,2-Distearoyl-sn-glycero-3-phosphocholine, and cholesterol), potassium chloride, monobasic potassium phosphate, sodium chloride, dibasic sodium phosphate dihydrate, and sucrose (Food and Drug Administration, 2021). In the contents of this vaccine, nor in any others, are there any microchips included.

Clinical Trials

There have been numerous unfounded claims about the clinical trials for various COVID-19 vaccines. People have come up with theories claiming that clinical trials were faked, rushed, or covered up adverse reactions and deaths. In one Facebook post, people were warned against participating in vaccine trials in India as the Chinese government was using them as guinea pigs after running out of laboratory monkeys. In regard to the trials being rushed, it is true that the development and emergency authorization of vaccines in such a short period of time is unprecedented. Under normal circumstances, vaccines may take up to 10 years to be approved. However, this is usually due to a lack of funding and other hurdles. With the COVID-19 vaccines, funding was not an issue. The rapid development of these vaccines was also the result of the collective work of a large number of scientists and volunteers. As well, there was pre-existing technology and knowledge about other coronaviruses which was used as a foundation for researchers in their fight against SARS-CoV-2. Clinical trials for the COVID-19 vaccines were also monitored by multiple countries where safety reports were provided to regulators. The FDA also monitors and reprimands companies and firms which promote fraudulent COVID-19 vaccines and provide false data.

Killer Vaccines and Overpopulation

Of the many vaccine-related conspiracies that have gone viral since the start of the pandemic, one of the most concerning is the claim that the COVID-19 vaccines were created to reduce overpopulation and find a zero carbon solution to climate change. Believers and perpetuators of this theory commonly refer to a Bill Gates quote from a 2010 TED talk where he states: "The world today has 6.8 billion people. That's headed up to about nine billion. Now, if we do a really great job on new vaccines, health care, reproductive health services, we could lower that by, perhaps, 10 or 15 percent".

Taken out of context, the quote has been misconstrued as Gates suggesting that vaccines will be used to kill people. However, within the context of the full TED talk, titled Innovating to Zero, it becomes clear that Gates is simply expressing that if healthcare and vaccination rates are improved, then population growth will stabilize. Indeed, as healthcare is improved in countries, infant mortality decreases and as a consequence, birth rates also decrease (Raivio, 1990). This is because if children are dying, parents tend to have more offspring in order to ensure that at least some survive (Raivio, 1990). For example, a study of Bangladeshi families found that in a family where no children had died, the average total fertility rate (TFR) of 2.6 children (Raivio, 1990). In families where one child had died, there was an average TFR of 4.7 children (Raivio, 1990). And in families where two children had died, there was an average TFR of 6.2 children (Raivio, 1990). With this context and explanation, it becomes clear the viral Bill Gates quote is harmless and vaccines will not be used to kill anyone.

Solutions

In an attempt to combat the flurry of misinformation that is posted to the internet every day, social media platforms have made significant efforts to crack down on posts that contain misleading information about COVID-19 or vaccines. As of May 2021, Facebook reported that it had taken down 16 million posts due to violation of its misinformation policy for COVID-19 and vaccines (Sriskandarajah, 2021). Another 167 million posts had been given warnings after failing to pass fact-checking (Sriskandarajah, 2021). On YouTube, over 900,000 videos containing misinformation about COVID-19 were removed, 30,000 of which were only about vaccines (Sriskandarajah, 2021). The popular social media app, TikTok, also has a policy that prohibits and removes COVID-19 related content that is false or misleading. This includes anti-vaccine misinformation. On both TikTok and Instagram, anti-vaccine hashtags are not autocompleted. Instead, trying to search up anti-vaccine content leads to a suggestion to redirect the user to a reliable source of information, such as the Public Health Agency of Canada or the World Health Organization. Despite these efforts, the Center for Countering Digital Hate revealed that 95% of COVID-19 and vaccine related misinformation reported to them is not taken action against by social media platforms (Sriskandarajah, 2021).

Other efforts to combat COVID-19 misinformation have included a White House national COVID-19 response proposal which included plans for rapid detection of misinformation and a "mass education campaign" to provide people with accurate information on vaccines as well as their importance (Sriskandarajah, 2021). In early July, president Joe Biden introduced an initiative to encourage Americans to get vaccinated by going door-to-door through communities. The CDC has also begun to create a system to monitor public health misinformation. As well, The Virality Project is another initiative built by a coalition of research entities in the United States in order to "detect, analyze, and respond to incidents of false and misleading narratives related to COVID-19 vaccines across online ecosystems, enabling civil society and health communicators to ultimately mitigate the impact of narratives which might otherwise undermine the public's confidence in the safety of evidence-based policies in the United States"

(The Virality Project, n.d.). As well, there has been an increasing emphasis on finding trustworthy sources for public health related information rather than blindly trusting social media content from unofficial sources. The CDC website has a page dedicated to this where they suggest sources for credible vaccine information.

Conclusion

Vaccine hesitancy is not always unreasonable. Many people hold valid concerns and questions regarding vaccines and should not be labelled conspiracy theorists or anti-vaxxers for wanting to be properly informed. However, there are occasions where skepticism and mistrust is taken in the wrong direction and leads one down a slippery slope of fear and conspiracies, where logic is abandoned. Due to the detrimental effects that conspiracy theories can have on public health, it is of utmost importance to continue to try and combat misinformation. Whether it be through government led initiatives or social media platform content restrictions, the reduction of conspiracies and a shift towards fact-checking and analytical thinking is something that will benefit all of humanity.

Chapter 11: Limitations And Risks Of Vaccines

Further reasons for the general public to have vaccine hesitancy are the risks that come with receiving a vaccination, as well as how the availability of vaccines can be very inconsistent, especially when considering the regions they are being administered in and the socioeconomic status of the people receiving the vaccine. In December of 2019, the novel coronavirus disease was discovered in China before spreading throughout the world, quickly becoming a global pandemic, and leading the World Health Organization to declare a global health emergency. Despite vaccine development being a lengthy process, being able to take approximately ten to fifteen years to complete, grand efforts to develop a vaccine that will combat COVID-19 has made the process go a lot quicker than what most researchers and citizens are accustomed to.

On March 30, 2020, the United States Department of Health and Human Services (HHS) started Operation Warp Speed (OWS) to commence the development of a coronavirus vaccine, Moderna then proceeded to release their initial clinical trial data from phases one and two on July 14, while Pfizer did the same on August 12, though this company did not take part in Operation Warp Speed. This rapid progress has left many feeling suspicious and questioning whether a vaccine is truly being developed despite the numerous explanations that a COVID vaccine needs to be discovered as the healthcare systems were severely overwhelmed at the time. This chapter will explore the limits and risks that cause citizens to be hesitant to receive a vaccine, especially referring to the coronavirus vaccines.

What are the risks of taking a vaccine?
Upon receiving a vaccine, the body can react in several ways due to the fact that it is attempting to adjust to the new substance entering the body. The three most common reactions are the side effects stemming from the vaccine itself, allergic reactions, and finally, reactions induced by the stress experienced by those who are fearful of needles and vaccines.

Side effects derived from the vaccine
The human body's natural response when dealing with a substance that it has never directly interacted with before is to reject it. Similarly to other medications, the body will try to reject anything foreign that enters it, which will result in side effects that can cause pain and can be visible.

Usually, side effects experienced upon obtaining a vaccine consist of:

> *"-symptoms at the injection site, such as:*
> - *pain*
> - *redness*
> - *swelling*
> - *flu-like symptoms, such as:*
>   - ◊ *chills*
>   - ◊ *fatigue*
>   - ◊ *joint pain*
>   - ◊ *headache*
>   - ◊ *mild fever*

◊   *muscle aches" (Canada, 2011, para. 6-7).*

Side effects derived from allergic reactions

Anaphylaxis is an extremely severe allergic reaction that can occur within either seconds or minutes of the time a person has been exposed to an allergen in the item(s) they are allergic to. The immune system will attack the body immediately, "the blood pressure drops suddenly and your airways narrow, blocking breathing. Signs and symptoms include a rapid, weak pulse; a skin rash; and nausea and vomiting. Common triggers include certain foods, some medications, insect venom and latex" (Mayo Clinic, 2019, para. 2). There is some chance to be allergic to certain substances in a vaccine, thus leading to a reaction shortly afterwards. The reaction, however, can be immediately treated with a dose of epinephrine in order to reverse the allergic reaction.

Side effects derived from stress

Trypanophobia is a very common fear across all age groups, and can be quite severe in some cases. Anxiety catalyzed by either getting a vaccine or the anticipation of getting a vaccine can affect how one reacts before, after, and during the time the vaccine is being administered. This level of unease from awaiting a vaccination can cause a drastic drop in blood pressure, sweating, irregular breathing, excessive sweating, numbness in the body, especially the face, hands, and feet, and finally, lightheadedness or dizziness that can cause the patient to faint either during or after their vaccinations.

What are the risks of not taking a vaccine?

The purpose of receiving a vaccine is for an individual and/ or individuals to obtain immunity to the microorganism that they are having enter their body. This will therefore "in some cases, … give lifelong immunity, but in other cases, the vaccination must be repeated at regular intervals" (Act For Libraries, 2017, para. 1). By doing so, the individual that obtains immunization also obtains protection for themselves as well as their loved ones and other people surrounding them; it provides protection from potentially fatal diseases. Therefore, when an individual decides that they do not wish to receive an immunization, they are putting themselves, as well as their community, at a higher risk of contracting a vaccine-preventable disease. For example, if a vaccine-preventable disease causes an outbreak in the community, those who have not been vaccinated are more susceptible to the symptoms endured by those who have contracted the disease.

What difficulties have been encountered during the development of the COVID-19 vaccine?

One difficulty that was encountered as the COVID-19 vaccine was being developed was during the pre-clinical trials. Due to the fact that most animals do not contract the SARS-CoV-2 infection, preclinical vaccine testing against the disease was difficult. Having no animals to test the vaccine on prevents researchers from testing it on humans, as the interactions of the vaccine with animals with similar DNA to humans must be evaluated before having humans as test subjects (Pouton, 2020).

Another issue with the development of the COVID-19 vaccine is the manner in which it is being distributed. While some nations have been able to easily administer the vaccine, other nations have been struggling with having enough COVID-19 doses in stock. The creation and distribution of vaccines is quite complicated, which is why there has been shortages in terms of vaccine deliveries across certain nations. Also, commencing vaccine production is not something that can occur spontaneously, as "vaccines are protected by intellectual property laws, and only facilities licensed by the pharmaceutical companies that own the patents are permitted to make them" (Sheldon, 2021, para. 21). COVID-19 Vaccines Global Access is an initiative backed by the World Health Organization that is meant to support the countries that do not have enough of the coronavirus vaccine, and though it "had pledged to deliver 231 million doses to 142 countries by the end of May this year, [it] was only able to ship 80 million" (Sheldon, 2021, para. 15).

What are the possibilities of contracting the COVID-19 disease upon receiving a dose of the vaccine?
One of the greatest causes for vaccine hesitancy when it comes to receiving the coronavirus vaccine is the fear that the disease could be contracted upon vaccination. Due to the severity of the coronavirus global pandemic, the production of COVID-19 vaccines had been hastened. As vaccines typically take several years to develop, many citizens are not very trusting towards the coronavirus vaccines being produced as they question their quality.

What does the efficacy rate of a vaccine tell us?
When most people hear of a vaccine's efficacy rate, they mistake it for how well the vaccine works once administered to the general public, which is defined by vaccine effectiveness. Vaccine efficacy describes how much less of a risk there is to contract the disease being treated. In other words, it is "the percentage reduction in a disease in a group of people who received a vaccination in a clinical trial" (Ryan,

2021, para. 5).

The rarity of breakthrough cases

Upon studying how the COVID-19 vaccines are interacting with people in the real world, any fault found has been very minimal:

> *"Two studies published March 23 in The New England Journal of Medicine suggest that breakthrough cases are very rare among the fully vaccinated. One study found that just 4 of 8,121 employees at the University of Texas Southwestern Medical Center in Dallas tested positive for coronavirus after being fully vaccinated. The other found that just 7 of 14,990 California health care workers tested positive two weeks after their second dose.*
>
> *In both studies, the chance of infection after full vaccination was about 0.05 percent. The authors noted that the study findings are even more remarkable considering participants were likely to have a higher risk of exposure than average people because they work in health care settings. What's more, they were tested during a post-holiday surge of cases." (Crouch, 2021. Para. 16-17).*

What are some causes for a breakthrough case?

One straightforward reason for a breakthrough case to occur post-vaccination is due to the potentially incorrect manner in which the vaccine is administered. A vaccine can be incorrectly handled in several ways, such as not providing the patient with a full dose, the vaccine being injected into the incorrect part of the arm, or if the vials have not been kept at their required temperatures.

A weakened immune system can change how a person reacts to the vaccine they receive. A patient could be taking medications that would weaken their immune system, such as chemotherapy treatments for cancer, or prednisone for pneumonia. This therefore hinders their body's interaction with the vaccine once it enters their system.

Another reason for there to be issues with breakthrough cases after receiving the COVID-19 vaccine is due to the new coronavirus strains and variants. Although earlier data suggests that the COVID-19 vaccines available should be able to provide protection against any new strains or variants of the disease, there is still a possibility for either a strain or variant to not be affected by the treatment of the vaccine.

Why do we need two doses of the coronavirus vaccine?
Another cause for speculation of the coronavirus vaccines is the fact that two doses are required in order to be considered fully vaccinated. The quality of the coronavirus vaccine is already being questioned due to how quickly they have been developed, therefore having to receive the vaccine twice stirs a lot of suspicion in those who do not place a lot of trust in the healthcare system.

What is the difference between the first and second dose of the COVID-19 vaccine?
The purpose of the first dose is to prepare the immune system and give it time to recognize the foreign substance entering the patient's body. The second dose allows the body to "practice" its resistance against the disease. Studies have shown that the reason two doses are required to combat

coronavirus is that "the Pfizer-BioNTech and Moderna vaccines provoke a relatively weak immune response when given as just one dose. However, there was a stronger immune response when a second dose was added" (Seladi-Schulman, 2021, para.12).

Should people receive both doses of the COVID-19 vaccine?

Many people believe that since the coronavirus vaccines are highly effective fourteen days or more upon receiving the first dose, obtaining the second dose of the COVID-19 vaccine is not necessary at all. Also, everyone receiving only one dose will inevitably allow more people to have access to the vaccine, leading to more vaccinations. Therefore, the coronavirus vaccines' effectiveness and availability no longer need to be of concern to the general public. However, organizations within the healthcare sector, such as the Food and Drug Administration, recommend obtaining both doses of the COVID-19 vaccine. The vaccines were released for public use after testing the dosing schedule currently being used in the clinical trials. Therefore, the coronavirus vaccines have been designed to be administered in two doses in order to be fully effective.

The following chapter discusses how the world's experience with the coronavirus pandemic and COVID-19 vaccines will influence medicine in the future. Is it possible to repurpose existing medications? If so, how can we go about doing that?

Chapter 12: The Future Of Vaccines

"With every new vaccine development, vaccinologists gain a deeper understanding of the immune system on a cellular and molecular level and of host-pathogen interactions" (Gerberding & Haynes, 2021, p. 396).

When Canadians unite again and COVID-19 news discussions become replaced by the next impending issue, pharmaceutical companies will continue developing, assessing, and innovating vaccines. Vaccinologists continuously strive to innovate the effectiveness and accessibility of vaccines as they are unceasing in adapting the latest insights from technology (PMCPA, 2021). As discussed in earlier chapters at length, many approved vaccines from the past, including those used for measles (1963) and polio (1955), were created with attenuated viruses and without a profound understanding of viral pathogenesis (Gerberding & Haynes, 2021). Now, in 2021, over a year into the COVID-19 pandemic—and we're almost in need of a slight pinch at the thought of it— researchers emphasize how new vaccine designs hinge upon new technologies, considering these instruments "lead us to a deeper understanding of the immune system and of host-pathogen interactions" (Gerberding & Haynes, 2021, p. 396). Pondering that notion, we'd realize that in many instances throughout history—including in the stories shared in Chapter 1—technology played a chief role in the discovery and in overcoming diseases and viruses. Technology, a capability that transcends the human eye, enables scientists to accomplish the feats our vaccine pioneers aspired to. Throughout this book, we learned about the many facets of vaccine development: the vaccine pioneers, the many forms of vaccines, how active agents produce lasting immunity to novel antigens, the events that left trauma, and even the process behind clinical testing and marketing vaccines. But above all, we hope to have relayed this to our readers: While today's viral, subunit, RNA, polysaccharide inoculations, and so forth, may be more advanced, a feat to our traditional (inactivated) vaccines, a commonality persists through time, humanity's sustenance of health and life depends upon vaccine developments (Ulmer & Liu, 2021; Branswell, 2021). Disease is inevitable, and it's a constant tyrant in need of overcoming for our survival.

As was likely said during past outbreaks, the pandemic (presently COVID-19) has reminded us of why the world necessitates vaccines. To list the determinants of COVID-19 alone, the morbidity, the 4 million lives lost as of July of 2021, the economic setback of 10.3 trillion in GDP in 2020, which has been likened to the Great Depression and the two world wars, showcased to us all how destructive the virus is, and, ultimately, the shining armour of the vaccines during this crisis (Ulmer & Liu, 2021; Worldometer, 2021, "COVID-19 Coronavirus Pandemic"; Kong, 2021). It is important to note that if scientists weren't actively working on RNA vaccines for 30 years and presently tackling mutations, the economic setback and the number of deaths would likely brink to that of the Black Plague or the Spanish flu (Ulmer & Liu, 2021). To be exact, if COVID-19 began five years ago, our RNA vaccines wouldn't be of the maturity needed to be rapidly used (Branswell, 2021).

What COVID-19 Taught Us About Vaccines
As stated by vaccine consultants Ulmer & Liu (2021):

> *The impact of the SARS-CoV-2 pandemic in terms of lives lost, morbidity, and depression of the global economy has demonstrated the importance of vaccines. We have been reminded that despite all the advances in medicine and other technologies, vaccines appear to be the only means of both protecting lives and health, and returning society to some degree of normalcy. (p. 1)*

During this unbearably long but short length of time, the COVID-19 pandemic has provided scientists with invaluable information about coronaviruses and delivery. The first insight, as stressed by John Mascola, the head of the National Institute of Allergy and Infectious Diseases Vaccine Research Center, producing a vaccine—in fact, six—wasn't a mere fluke (Branswell, 2021). That's because fortunately, the 2002-2003 SARS outbreak and 2012 camel coronavirus (MERS) alerted scientists to begin creating vaccines for coronaviruses. As demonstrated, it's crucial that epidemiologists monitor for new outbreaks and swiftly implement preventive measures.

The second insight, and an example to draw upon for future reference, involves the Trump administration's handling of funding (Branswell, 2021). If only Canada adapted their approach. Rather than funding one or two projects, the U.S. president poured into several different projects, all of which were developing different types of modern vaccines. Out of the six projects funded, two of them focused on messenger RNA vaccines, another two on viral vectors, and the remaining two on protein-based vaccines. As of June 30th, 2021, 5 out of 6 of the projects were successful and led to a vaccine or will soon be made into a vaccine. In hindsight, the act of dispersing funding, which proved successful, was rooted in mindfulness for how "more projects fail than succeed" (Branswell, 2021, para. 10). That's a quintessential example of strategic emergency planning.

If only the same success could be attributed to these next hurdles, containing a myriad of intricate problems that permeated across North America. Two of those obstacles involve accessibility and distribution, hurdles in which scientists promise to clear in the future. What do scientists propose as a fix for them? To start, vaccines only requiring administration once are under development. Apart from needing technologies for a one-time dose, they project a more powerful vaccine or packing that allows "for its contents [to be] released intermittently once it has been administered" is necessary (Australian Academy of Science, 2021, para. 3).

What were the specific issues with accessibility and distribution though? Let's elaborate. As anticipated, upon a vaccine being developed, the demand surpassed the supply available (Branswell, 2021). America, much like Canada, would have to choose who would first receive the jab. Officials agreed essential workers, such as nurses or those who conduct critical operations, were first in line. Selecting who was eligible, or an essential worker, was no small task though, and it created much scheduling havoc in America. Conflict in distribution was feeding from the trough of another giant though. In other words, the issue ran deeper than mere scheduling. Additionally, the cold storage required, which was to ensure the vaccines' potency, limited the number of jabs produced for distribution to only 1,000 doses. Thus, fewer people could be vaccinated at once and an unbearable wait time, much like rain clouds during a drought, would loom over people's heads until so; the preventive was discovered, but not exactly obtainable. That's an issue.

When the next pandemic rolls around (as much as we almost pass a kidney stone at the sounds of it), it will, or should, be a smoother process. Our leaders and scientists are working to find a solution to these post-development issues, and they have been for years. As best described by The College of Physicians of Philadelphia (2018), "the future of immunization depends on the success of medical research for vaccines that are simpler to administer, will survive transport even without refrigeration, and will provide a more substantial and long-lasting immune response" (para. 16).

Overall, this course of action sounds feasible and a way to hack the problem at the root.

We're All Wondering—Will Future Vaccine Developments Accelerate?

Modern vaccines are quickening in their development but scientists caution against the thinking that instantaneous or drive-thru vaccines are underway (Boyle, 2021). Since the COVID-19 vaccines were created in eleven months, some speculate that future vaccine developments will require less and less time in the future (Ulmer & Liu, 2021). Although scientists hypothesize that future RNA vaccines will be developed within four or even three months, which is considerably shorter than COVID's 11 months, the vaccines are still a work-in-progress (Boyle, 2021). We haven't crossed the finish line just yet. As mentioned in Chapter 5, once RNA vaccines are perfected, researchers will simply alter the genetic sequencing encoded. Adding to the advantages of RNA vaccines, which are slowly gaining the support of researchers and pharmaceutical companies, the cost of producing vaccines would be reduced. Another bonus, no one would ever present a painstaking 10-year vaccine development plan in boardrooms. Previously struggling to gain funding for mRNA research, scientists hope the success of Pfizer (95%) and Moderna (94.1%) will change that narrative. Research, social, financial, and political factors play a big role in vaccine developments (Boyle, 2021). Also, I'd like to supersize my burger, fries, and vaccine, please.

What to Expect in the Future for Vaccines

Other than future developments in mRNA vaccines for several types of cancers, tumour cells, cystic fibrosis, Hepatitis B, malaria, and so forth, another vaccine design will soon hold the public's attention (Boyle, 2021). They're called DNA vaccines. DNA vaccines, often referred to as third-generation vaccines, haven't been discussed at length in this book, considering only one of its kind was produced late into the COVID pandemic (Cuffari, 2021). Only at the beginning of July in 2021 was ZyCoV-D announced the fifth vaccine available in India (HT Correspondent, 2021). More news coverage will likely emerge as it's the world's first DNA vaccine ever approved. Caffari, a former anticancer therapy researcher, explains the function of DNA vaccines (2021):

> Like any other type of vaccine, DNA vaccines induce an adaptive immune response. The basic working principle behind any DNA vaccine involves the use of a DNA plasmid that encodes for a protein that originated from the pathogen in which the vaccine will be targeted. (para. 8)

Essentially, DNA vaccines (including RNA) are similar to traditional vaccines in that they "induce an adaptive immune response." But, a difference lies in how DNA and RNA vaccines work (Hensley, 2020). While all vaccines seek to cultivate immunity in the human body, genetic vaccines encode a protein from the pathogen. Cuffari explains further, "DNA vaccines . . . use engineered DNA to induce an immunologic response in the host against bacteria, parasites, viruses, and potentially cancer" (2021, para. 1). As traditional vaccines use a weakened form of a virus or bacteria, "DNA and RNA vaccines use part of the virus' genetic code to stimulate an immune response . . . In other words, they carry the genetic instructions for the host's cells to make antigens" (Hensley, 2020, "Key Takeaways"-para. 5).

The Differences Between RNA and DNA Vaccines
DNA vaccines differ from RNA vaccines in that "the virus' genetic information is transmitted to another molecule called the messenger RNA (mRNA) (Hensley, 2020, para. 9). RNA vaccines are essentially one step ahead of DNA vaccines. Additionally, DNA vaccines deliver the message through a "small electrical pulse, which literally pushes the message into the cell" (Hensley, 2020, para. 11). One advantage to DNA vaccines is that they remain stable in warmer temperatures. Aside from India's emergency authorized ZyCoV-D (66.6%), other DNA and RNA vaccines are currently in clinical trials in the United States (HT Correspondent, 2021; Hensley, 2020).

Can We Expect RNA and DNA Vaccines to Dominate the Industry?
Since COVID-19 emerged, viral-vector and nucleic-acid-based vaccines have been the focus of preventive discussions (Immunisation Advisory Centre, 2020). And,

while genetic vaccines are the latest design scientists are working on, previous forms will continue to be administered (Branswell, 2021). Genetic vaccines have demonstrated their effectiveness for pandemics and outbreaks, but they won't be the only form used moving forward (Boyle, 2021). With dealing with diverse pathogens and infectious agents, "the solutions will always be diverse. There's never going to be a single solution to every problem" (Boyle, 2021, para. 21). Considering they are new technologies, RNA and DNA vaccines are also still under scrutiny and will be for years to come (Branswell, 2021). Until then, who knows, perhaps a preventive for HIV will become available and, not too long after that, a therapeutic cancer vaccine or a Hepatitis B inoculation.

About the Authors

Mohathir Sheikh is an author and student completing his Bachelor of Commerce after-degree concentrating in Business Analytics. His passion to use data to make informed decisions has led to him creating a Discord group with his peers, where he shares daily market news and stock analysis. He holds a Bachelor of Health Sciences degree in Biomedical Sciences, in which he conducted a year-long thesis studying myelination in dorsal root ganglion and cortical neurons. Throughout the pandemic, he has published books on numerous topics that can be found on Amazon, Lulu, Google Scholar, and ResearchGate.

Fariha Khan is an author, artist, and graphic designer. After completion of her Bachelor of Science degree in Psychology, she hopes to attend medical school in Canada and later work as a clinical psychiatrist. Her interest in art and design has led her to work with AIC where she has collaborated with teams of student writers to develop cover designs and interiors for their publications, publishing 10 books in both print and electronic format. The books can be found on Amazon, Lulu, Google Scholar, and ResearchGate.

Angela Kazmierczak is an author, communications specialist, and journalist. She holds a Bachelor's in Communication Studies and is currently studying Radio and Television. Into the early months of the COVID-19 pandemic, she and a team of AIC writers wrote the book, The Misinformation of COVID-19. To her, the book was a precursor to writing about the COVID-19 vaccines, since it was then she discovered preventive discussions are most prey to misinformation. Her other works can be found on Academia, Research Gate, Amazon, or on Google Scholar.

Yemariam Abebayehu is an author and spoken word poet. She is pursuing a Bachelor of Arts degree in Psychology and French Language and Literature, while also completing a certificate in French Translation Studies. A month before lockdown started, Yemariam released her debut poem anthology, Open Flame. It is a collection of poems organized in three stages under the common theme of allowing ourselves to display our most intense emotions, although doing so is frowned upon by society. Readers can find her anthology at the Blurb Bookstore.

References

Abu-Raddad, L. J., Chemaitelly, H., Butt, A. A. (2021). Effectiveness of the BNT162b2 Covid-19 Vaccine against the B.1.1.7 and B.1.351 Variants, The New England Journal of Medicine, DOI: 10.1056/NEJMc2104974

Accra, G. (2015, September 7). *Module 2: Vaccines and drugs* [PowerPoint slides]. Vaccine PV Fellowship. https://isoponline.org/wp-content/uploads/2015/10/DiffereNces-on-drugs-and-vaccines.pdf

Act For Libraries. (2017). What is the Purpose of Vaccines. Retrieved from Actforlibraries.org website: http://www.actforlibraries.org/what-is-the-purpose-of-vaccines/

Ada, G. (2005). Overview of vaccines and vaccination. *Molecular Biotechnology,* 29(3), 255–272. https://doi.org/10.1385/MB:29:3:255

Aiello, A., Farzaneh, F., Candore, G., Caruso, C., Davinelli, S., Gambino, C. M., Ligotti, M. E., Zareian, N., & Accardi, G. (2019). Immunosenescence and Its Hallmarks: How to Oppose Aging Strategically? A Review of Potential Options for Therapeutic Intervention. Frontiers in immunology, 10, 2247. https://doi.org/10.3389/fimmu.2019.02247

Alzheimer Europe - Research - Understanding dementia research - Clinical trials - Types of clinical trials. (2016). Retrieved May 18, 2021, from Alzheimer-europe.org website: https://www.alzheimer-europe.org/Research/ Understanding-dementia-research/Clinical-trials/Types-of-clinical-trials

Ammer, C. (2013). Where there's smoke, there's fire. In *The Free Dictionary.* Retrieved July 22, 2021, from https:// idioms.thefreedictionary.com/where+there%27s+smok e%2C+there%27s+fire

Anderson, R. M., Vegvari, C., Truscott, J., & Collyer, B. S. (2020). Challenges in creating herd immunity to SARS-CoV-2 infection by mass vaccination. *The Lancet,* 396(10263), 1614– 1616. https://doi.org/10.1016/S0140-6736(20)32318-7

Andreano, E., D'Oro, U., Rappuoli, R., & Finco, O. (2019). Vaccine evolution and its application to fight modern threats. *Frontiers in Immunology,* 10(1722), 1-5. https://doi. org/10.3389/fimmu.2019.01722

Arsenault, A. (2020, December 22). A Timeline of COVID-19 (Coronavirus). Retrieved July 9, 2021, from Verywell Health website: https://www.verywellhealth.com/coronavirus-covid-19-timeline-4798671

Augustyn, A. (n.d.). Germ theory. In *Encyclopaedia Britannica.* Retrieved May 29, 2021, from https://www.britannica.com/ science/germ-theory

Australian Academy of Science. (2021). What does the future hold for vaccination? http://www.science.org.au/education/immunisation-climate-change-genetic-modifi cation/science-immunisation/5-what-does-future

Badiani, A. A., Patel, J. A., Ziolkowski, K., & Nielsen, F. (2020). Pfizer: The miracle vaccine for COVID-19?. Public Health in Practice, 1, 100061. https://doi.org/10.1016/j.puhip.2020.100061

Balfour, H. (2020, March 27). *Remdesivir most promising COVID-19 drug, say researchers.* Drug Target Review. https://www.drugtargetreview.com/news/58608/remdesivir-most-promising-covid-19-drug-say-researchers/

Baraniuk, C. (2021). How long does covid-19 immunity last?, BMJ, 373, doi: https://doi.org/10.1136/bmj.n1605

BBC News. (2021). Coronavirus: WHO chief criticises 'shocking' global vaccine divide. Retrieved June 19, 2020 from https://www.bbc.com/news/world-56698854

Beusekom, M. V. (2021). Disparities in US COVID vaccine distribution spotlighted. Retrieved June 20, 2021 from https://www.cidrap.umn.edu/news-perspective/2021/05/disparities-us-covid-vaccine-distribution-spotlighted

Beusekom, M. V. (2021). Pfizer, AstraZeneca COVID-19 vaccines may offer high efficacy in elderly, Center for Infectious Disease Research and Policy. Retrieved June 21, 2021 from https://www.cidrap.umn.edu/news-perspective/2021/03/pfizer-astrazeneca-covid-19-vaccines-may-offer-high-efficacy-elderly.

Billingsley, A. (2020, April 30). *The novel coronavirus: What are novel viruses, and how do they impact public health?* GoodRx. https://www.goodrx.com/blog/what-does-novel-coronavirus-mean-science-medical-definition/

Biography.com Editors (2021, May 28). Louis Pasteur. In *A&E Television Networks Biography.* Retrieved May 28, 2021, from https://www.biography.com/scientist/louis-pasteur

Biology Dictionary Editors. (2017, May 15). Germ theory definition. In *Biology Dictionary.* Retrieved May 29, 2021, from https://biologydictionary.net/germ-theory/

Boni, M.F., Lemey, P., Jiang, X., Lam, T. T.Y., Perry B. W., Castoe, T. A., Rambaut, A., Robertson, D. L. (2020). Evolutionary origins of the SARS-CoV-2 sarbecovirus lineage responsible for the COVID-19 pandemic. Nat Microbiol 5, 1408–1417. https://doi.org/10.1038/s41564-020-0771-4

Boylston, A. (2012). The origins of inoculation. *Journal of the Royal Society of Medicine, 105(7),* 309-313. https://doi.org/10.1258%2Fjrsm.2012.12k044
Retrieved May 29, 2021, from https://biologydictionary.net/germ-theory/

Branswell, H. (2021, June 30). 12 lessons COVID-19 taught us about developing vaccines during a pandemic. STAT. http://www.statnews.com/2021/06/30/12-lessons-covid-19-developing-vaccines/

Brock, R. (2021). Is it Ethical to Uphold Vaccine Patents during a Global Shortage? https://www.scu.edu/ethics/healthcare-ethics-blog/is-it-ethical-to-uphold-vaccine-patents-during-a-global-shortage/

Brodie, C. (2017, September 11). Vaccines have killed off these deadly diseases. Retrieved June 2, 2021, from World Economic Forum website: https://www.weforum.org/agenda/2017/09/vaccines-have-killed-off-these-deadly-diseases/

Brothers, W. (2020, December 3). A Timeline of COVID-19 Vaccine Development. Retrieved July 9, 2021, from BioSpace website: https://www.biospace.com/article/a-timeline-of-covid-19-vaccine-development/

Brown, K. V. (2021, March 14). Bloomberg - Are you a robot? Retrieved July 22, 2021, from www.bloomberg.com website: https://www.bloomberg.com/news/newsletters/2021-03-14/what-does-vaccine-efficacy-really-mean#:~:text=%E2%80%9CEfficacy%20is%20a%20measure%20of%20relative%20reduction%20in

Burger, L., Nair, A. (2021). AstraZeneca, Pfizer vaccines effective against Delta COVID-19 variants: study. Retrieved June 27, 2021 from https://www.ctvnews.ca/health/coronavirus/astrazeneca-pfizer-vaccines-effective-against-delta-covid-19-variants-study-1.5482427

Calina, D., Docea, A. O., Petrakis, D., Egorov, A. M., Ishmukhamerov, A. A., Gabibov, A. G.,Shtilman, M. I., Kostoff, R., Carvalho, F., Vinceti, M., Spandidos, D. A., & Tstatsakis, A. (2020, May 6). Towards effective COVID-19 vaccines: Updates,
perspectives and challenges. *International Journal of Molecular Medicine,* 46(1), 3-16. https://doi.org/10.3892/ijmm.2020.4596

Campbell, L. (2021). Debunking COVID-19 Vaccine Myths Spreading on Parent Facebook Groups. Retrieved July 12, 2021 from https://www.healthline.com/health-news/debunking-covid-19-vaccine-myths-spreading-on-parent-facebook-groups

Cameron, C. E., & Lukehart, S. A. (2014). Current status of syphilis vaccine development: Need, challenges, prospects. *Vaccine, 32*(14), 1602–1609. https://doi.org/10.1016/j.vaccine.2013.09.053

Canada, H. (2011, January 26). Regulating vaccines for human use in Canada. Retrieved May 21, 2021, from aem website: https://www.canada.ca/en/health-canada/services/drugs-health-products/biologics-radiopharmaceuticals-genetic-therapies/activities/fact-sheets/regulation-vaccines-human-canada.html

Canada, H. (2020, December 8). Vaccine development and approval in Canada. Retrieved May 19, 2021, from aem website: https://www.canada.ca/en/health-canada/services/drugs-health-products/covid19-industry/drugs-vaccines-treatments/vaccines/development-approval-infographic.html

Cao, Y., & Gao, G. F. (2021). mRNA vaccines: A matter of delivery. EClinicalMedicine, 32, 100746. https://doi.org/10.1016/j.eclinm.2021.100746

Cardona, G. (n.d.). Devanagari writing system. In *Encyclopaedia Britannica.* Retrieved June 9, 2021, from https://www.britannica.com/topic/Devanagari

Carfì, A., Bernabei, R., Landi, F., & Gemelli Against COVID-19 Post-Acute Care Study Group (2020). Persistent Symptoms in Patients After Acute COVID-19. JAMA, 324(6), 603–605. https://doi.org/10.1001/jama.2020.12603

Catanzaro, M., Fagiani, F., Racchi, M., Corsini, E., Govoni, S., Lanni, C. (2020). Immune response in COVID-19: addressing a pharmacological challenge by targeting pathways triggered by SARS-CoV-2. Signal Transduction and Targeted Therapy, 5, 84. https://doi.org/10.1038/s41392-020-0191-1

Centers for Disease Control and Prevention. (n.d.). Autism and Vaccines. Retrieved July 3, 2021 from https://www.cdc.gov/vaccinesafety/concerns/autism.html

Centers for Disease Control and Prevention. (2021). *COVID-19, Frequently Asked Questions.* Retrieved May 22, 2021 from: https://www.cdc.gov/coronavirus/2019-ncov/faq.html.

Centers for Disease Control and Prevention. (2021). *Guidance for Unvaccinated People, Protect Yourself.* Retrieved May 22, 2021 from: https://www.cdc.gov/coronavirus/2019-ncov/prevent-getting-sick/prevention.html.

Centers for Disease Control and Prevention. (2021). *Johnson & Johnson's Janssen COVID-19 Vaccine Overview and Safety.* Retrieved June 12, 2021 from https://www.cdc.gov/coronavirus/2019-ncov/vaccines/different-vaccines/janssen.html

Centers for Disease Control and Prevention. (2021). *Older Adults.* Retrieved June 21, 2021 from https://www.cdc.gov/coronavirus/2019-ncov/need-extra-precautions/older-adults.html

Centers for Disease Control and Prevention. (2021). *Moderna COVID-19 Vaccine Storage and Handling Summary.* Retrieved June 12, 2021 from https://www.cdc.gov/vaccines/covid-19/info-by-product/moderna/downloads/storage-summary.pdf

Centers for Disease Control and Prevention. (2021). *Pfizer-BioNTech COVID-19 Vaccine Storing and Handling Summary.* Retrieved June 12, 2021 from https://www.cdc.gov/vaccines/covid-19/info-by-product/pfizer/downloads/storage-summary.pdf

Centers for Disease Control and Prevention. (2021). *Potential Treatments.* Retrieved May 23, 2021 from: https://www.cdc.gov/coronavirus/2019-ncov/your-health/treatments-for-severe-illness.html.

Centers for Disease Control and Prevention. (2021). *SARS-CoV-2 Variant Classifications and Definitions.* Retrieved June 6, 2021 from https://www.cdc.gov/coronavirus/2019-ncov/variants/variant-info.html

Centers for Disease Control and Prevention. (2021, January 26). *Malaria.*
https://www.cdc.gov/malaria/about/faqs.html

Centers for Disease Control and Prevention. (2021). *Older Adults and COVID-19.* Retrieved May 23, 2021 from: https://www.cdc.gov/coronavirus/2019-ncov/need-extra-precautions/older-adults.html.

Centers for Disease Control and Prevention. (2021). *Origin of Smallpox.*
http://www.cdc.gov/smallpox/symptoms/index.html

Centers for Disease Control and Prevention. (2020). *Principles of vaccination. U.S. Department of Health and Human Services.* https://www.cdc.gov/vaccines/pubs/pinkbook/prinvac.html

Centers for Disease Control and Prevention. (2021). *Risk for COVID-19 Infection, Hospitalization, and Death.* Retrieved May 23, 2021 from: https://www.cdc.gov/coronavirus/2019-ncov/covid-data/investigations-discovery/hospitalization-death-by-age.html.

Centers for Disease Control and Prevention. (2019). *Risks of Delaying or Skipping Vaccines.* Retrieved July 8, 2021, from Centers for Disease Control and Prevention website: https://www.cdc.gov/vaccines/parents/why-vaccinate/risks-delaying-vaccines.html

Centers for Disease Control and Prevention. (2021). *SARS-CoV-2 Variant Classifications and Definitions.* Retrieved June 6, 2021 from https://www.cdc.gov/coronavirus/2019-ncov/variants/variant-info.html

Centers for Disease Control and Prevention. (2018). *Understanding how vaccines work. U.S. Department of Health and Human Services.* https://www.cdc.gov/vaccines/hcp/conversations/downloads/vacsafe-understand-color-office.pdf

Chowdhury, M. A., Hossain, N., Kashem, M. A., Shahid, M. A., & Alam, A. (2020). *Immune response in COVID-19: A review. Journal of infection and public health, 13*(11), 1619–1629. https://doi.org/10.1016/j.jiph.2020.07.001

Cirino, E. (2017). Trypanophobia: Test, Definition, and Causes. Retrieved July 8, 2021, from Healthline website: https://www.healthline.com/health/trypanophobia

Clem, A. S. (2011). Fundamentals of Vaccine Immunology. *Journal of Global Infectious Diseases, 3*(1), 73–78. https://doi.org/10.4103/0974-777X.77299

The College of Physicians of Philadelphia. (2021). *Chinese Smallpox Inoculation.* https://www.historyofvaccines.org/content/early-chinese-inoculation

The College of Physicians of Philadelphia. (2021). *History of Polio.* https://www.historyofvaccines.org/timeline/polio

The College of Physicians of Philadelphia. (2018, January 10). The future of Immunization. https://www. historyofvaccines.org/content/articles/future-immunization

The College of Physicians of Philadelphia. (2010). *Thomas Peebles, doctor who isolated measles virus, dies at 89.* https:// www.historyofvaccines.org/content/blog/thomas-peebles-doctor-who-isolated-measles-virus-dies-89

Coon, L. (2021, May 29). Why you need the second COVID-19 vaccine dose. Retrieved July 22, 2021, from OSF HealthCare Blog website: https://www.osfhealthcare.org/blog/why-you-need-the-second-covid-19-vaccine-dose/

Corona, A. (2020). *Disease Eradication: What Does It Take to Wipe out a Disease?* Corona. https://asm.org/Articles/2020/ March/Disease-Eradication-What-Does-It-Take-to-Wipe-out

Cox, L. S., Bellantuono, I., Lord, J. M., Sapey, E., Mannick, J. B., Partridge, L., Gordon, A. L., Steves, C. J, Witham, M. D. (2020). Tackling immunosenescence to improve COVID-19 outcomes and vaccine response in older adults, The Lancet Healthy Longevity, 1(2). DOI:https://doi.org/10.1016/S2666-7568(20)30011-8

Crouch, M. (2021, May 14). Can You Catch the Coronavirus After Getting Vaccinated? Retrieved from AARP website: https://www.aarp.org/health/conditions-treatments/info-2021/coronavirus-after-vaccination.html

Cuffari, B. (2021, March 17). *What is a DNA vaccine?* News-Medical.Net. https://www.news-medical.net/health/What-is-a-DNA-based-vaccine.aspx

Dalton, J. (2021, January 30). *Meat-eating creates risk of future pandemic that 'would make covid seem a dress rehearsal', scientists warn.* Independent. https://www.independent. ate-change/news/meat-coronavirus-pandemic-science-animals-b1794996.html

Darby, A. C., Hiscox, J. A. (2021). Covid-19: variants and vaccination, BMJ, 372, doi: https://doi.org/10.1136/bmj.n771 Davis, B. K., Wen, H., & Ting, J. P. (2011). The inflammasome NLRs in immunity, inflammation, and associated diseases. Annual review of immunology, 29, 707–735. https://doi. org/10.1146/annurev-immunol-031210-101405

Delany, I., Rappuoli, R., & De Gregorio, E. (2014). Vaccines for the 21st century. EMBO Molecular Medicine, 6(6), 708–720. https://doi.org/10.1002/emmm.201403876

Domingo, E. (1997). Rapid Evolution of Viral RNA Genomes, The Journal of Nutrition, (127)5, 958S–961S, https://doi. org/10.1093/jn/127.5.958S

Dos Santos W. G. (2020). Natural history of COVID-19 and current knowledge on treatment therapeutic options. Biomedicine & pharmacotherapy = Biomedecine & pharmacotherapie, 129, 110493. https://doi.org/10.1016/j. biopha.2020.110493

Douglas, K. M., Sutton, R. M., Cichocka, A. (2017). The Psychology of Conspiracy Theories, Current Directions in Psychological Science, 26(6), 538-542, DOI: https://doi. org/10.1177/0963721417718261

Douglas, R. G., & Samant, V. B. (2018). The Vaccine Industry. *Plotkin's Vaccines,* 41-50.e1. https://doi.org/10.1016/B978-0-323-35761-6.00004-3

Doughman, E. (2019). Global Vaccine Market Revenue to Reach $59.2 Billion by 2020. Pharmaceutical Processing World. https://www.pharmaceuticalprocessingworld.com/global-vaccine-market-revenue-to-reach-59-2-billion-by-2020/

Dove, A. (2005). Maurice Hilleman. *Nature Publishing Group, 11*(4), 52. https://www.nature.com/articles/nm1223.pdf

D'Souza, G., Dowdy, D. (2021). What is herd immunity and how can we achieve it with COVID-19?, John Hopkins Bloomberg School of Public Health. Retrieved May 30, 2021 from https://www.jhsph.edu/covid-19/articles/achieving-herd-immunity-with-covid19.html.

Duda, K. (2020, March 11). Antigenic drift and shift with the flu virus. *Verywell Health.* https://www.verywellhealth.com/what-are-antigenic-drift-and-shift-770400

Encyclopaedia Britannica editors. (2019). Tuskegee syphilis study | American history. In *Encyclopædia Britannica.* Retrieved from https://www.britannica.com/event/Tuskegee-syphilis-study

Encyclopaedia Britannica editors. (n.d.). Variolation. In *Encyclopaedia Britannica.* Retrieved May 16, 2021, from https://www.britannica.com/science/variolation

Esakandari, H., Nabi-Afjadi, M., Fakkari-Afjadi, J., Farahmandian, N., Miresmaeili, SM., Bahreini, E. (2020). A comprehensive review of COVID-19 characteristics, Biological Procedures Online, 22. doi: 10.1186/s12575-020-00128-2

European Medicines Agency. (2021). COVID-19 vaccine AstraZeneca: benefits still outweigh the risks despite possible link to rare blood clots with low blood platelets. Retrieved June 5, 2021 from https://www.ema.europa.eu/en/news/covid-19-vaccine-astrazeneca-benefits-still-outweigh-risks-despite-possible-link-rare-blood-clots

Facher, L. (2020, April 6). Fact-checking Trump's claims about hydroxychloroquine, the antimarlarial drug he's touting as a coronavirus treatment. *STAT News.* https://www.statnews.com/2020/04/06/trump-hydroxychloroquine-fact-check/

Faisst S. (1999). Propagation of viruses | Animal. Encyclopedia of Virology, 1408–1413. https://doi.org/10.1006/rwvi.1999.0236

Fleming, S. (2021, February 24). This is why you need that second COVID-19 vaccine dose, says WHO's Chief Scientist. Retrieved July 22, 2021, from World Economic Forum website: https://www.weforum.org/agenda/2021/02/second-vaccine-dose-covid-19-who/

Fontanet, A., Autran, B., Lina, B., Kieny, M. P., Karim, S. S. A., Sridhar, D. (2021). SARS-CoV-2 variants and ending the COVID-19 pandemic, The Lancet, (397)10278, 952-954, DOI:https://doi.org/10.1016/S0140-6736(21)00370-6

Food and Drug Administration. (n.d.). COVID-19 Vaccines. Retrieved June 19, 2021 from https://www.fda.gov/emergency-preparedness-and-response/coronavirus-disease-2019-covid-19/covid-19-vaccines

Food and Drug Administration. (2021). Know Your Treatment Options for COVID-19. Retrieved May 23, 2021 from: https://www.fda.gov/consumers/consumer-updates/know-your-treatment-options-covid-19#:~:text=The%20FDA%20has%20approved%20the,comparable%20to%20inpatient%20hospital%20care.

Food and Drug Administration. (2021). Pfizer-BioNTech COVID-19 Vaccine EUA Fact Sheet for Recipients and Caregivers. Retrieved July 12, 2021 from https://www.fda.gov/media/144414/download#:~:text=The%20Pfizer%2DBioNTech%20COVID%2D19%20Vaccine%20includes%20the%20following%20ingredients,)%2C%20potassium%20chloride%2C%20monobasic%20potassium

Food and Drug Administration. (2021). Pfizer-BioNTech COVID-19 Vaccine Frequently Asked Questions. Retrieved July 12, 2021 from https://www.fda.gov/emergency-preparedness-and-response/mcm-legal-regulatory-and-policy-framework/pfizer-biontech-covid-19-vaccine-frequently-asked-questions.

Food and Drug Administration. (2018, March 28). Smallpox. https://www.fda.gov/vaccines-blood-biologics/vaccines/smallpox

Forni, G., Mantovani, A., on behalf of the COVID-19 Commission of Accademia Nazionale dei Lincei, Rome. et al. COVID-19 vaccines: where we stand and challenges ahead. Cell Death Differ 28, 626–639 (2021). https://doi.org/10.1038/s41418-020-00720-9

Fox, M. (2021, July 22). British researchers find more evidence two-dose vaccines protect well against Delta variant of coronavirus. Retrieved July 22, 2021, from cnn website: https://cnnphilippines.com/world/2021/7/22/COVID-19-vaccine-Delta-variant.html

France-Presse, A. (2021). AstraZeneca Tests Booster Vaccine Against Beta Variant Of Covid. Retrieved June 27, 2021 from https://www.ndtv.com/world-news/coronavirus-astrazeneca-tests-booster-vaccine-against-beta-variant-of-covid-2473665

Gasparini, R., Panatto, D., Lai, P. L., & Amicizia, D. (2015). The "urban myth" of the association between neurological disorders and vaccinations. Journal of preventive medicine and hygiene, 56(1), E1–E8.

Gavi, The Vaccine Alliance. (2021). COVAX Vaccine Roll-out. Retrieved June 19, 2021 from https://www.gavi.org/covax-vaccine-roll-out

Gavriatopoulou, M., Korompoki, E., Fotiou, D., Ntanasis-Stathopoulos, I., Psaltopoulou, T., Kastritis, E., Terpos, E., & Dimopoulos, M. A. (2020). Organ-specific manifestations of COVID-19 infection. Clinical and experimental medicine, 20(4), 493–506. https://doi.org/10.1007/s10238-020-00648-x

Geddes, A. M. (2006). The history of smallpox. *Clinics in Dermatology*, 24(3), 152-157. https://doi.org/10.1016/j. clindermatol.2005.11.009

Gearon, E. (n.d.). Who was Lady Mary Wortley Montagu? *University of Oxford.* http://www.nationaltrust.org.uk/ features/who-was-lady-Mary-wortley-montagu

Gerberding, J. L., & Haynes, B. F. (2021). Vaccine innovations—past and future. *The New England Journal of Medicine, 384*(5), 393-396. doi:10.1056/NEJMp2029466

Gilman, L. (2018, June 8). Smallpox. In *Encyclopedia.com encyclopedia.* Retrieved May 15, 2021, from, https://www. encyclopedia.com/medicine/diseases-and-conditions /pathology/smallpox

Goodman, B. (2021). Why COVID Vaccines are Falsely Linked to Infertility. Retrieved July 13, 2021 from https://www. webmd.com/vaccines/covid-19-vaccine/news/20210112/ why-covid-vaccines-are-falsely-linked-to-infertility

Government of Canada. (2021). COVID-19 mRNA vaccines. Retrieved June 5, 2021 from https://www.canada.ca/en/ health-canada/services/drugs-health-products/covid19-industry/drugs-vaccines-treatments/vaccines/type-mrna. html

Government of Canada. (2021). AstraZeneca/COVISHIELD COVID-19 vaccine. Retrieved June 5, 2021 from https:// www.canada.ca/en/health-canada/services/drugs-health-products/covid19-industry/drugs-vaccines-treatments/ vaccines/astrazeneca.html

Government of Canada. (2021). Janssen COVID-19 vaccine. Retrieved June 5, 2021 from https://www.canada.ca/en/health-canada/services/drugs-health-products/covid19-industry/drugs-vaccines-treatments/vaccines/janssen.html

Government of Canada. (2021). Moderna COVID-19 vaccine. Retrieved June 5, 2021 from https://www.canada.ca/en/health-canada/services/drugs-health-products/covid19-industry/drugs-vaccines-treatments/vaccines/moderna.html

Government of Canada. (2021). Pfizer-BioNTech COVID-19 vaccine. Retrieved June 5, 2021 from https://www.canada.ca/en/health-canada/services/drugs-health-products/covid19-industry/drugs-vaccines-treatments/vaccines/pfizer-biontech.html

Government of Canada. (2021). Viral vector-based vaccines for COVID-19. Retrieved June 5, 2021 from https://www.canada.ca/en/health-canada/services/drugs-health-products/covid19-industry/drugs-vaccines-treatments/vaccines/type-viral-vector.html

Government of Canada. (2021). COVID-19: Main modes of transmission, How COVID-19 spreads. Retrieved May 21, 2021 from: https://www.canada.ca/en/public-health/services/diseases/2019-novel-coronavirus-infection/health-professionals/main-modes-transmission.html.

Government of Canada (2018). *Pertussis vaccine: Canadian Immunization Guide.* https://www.canada.ca/en/public-health/services/publications/healthy-living/canadian-immunization-guide-part-4-active-vaccines/page-15-pertussis-vaccine.html

Government of Canada. (2018, October 10). *Poliomyelitis (Polio): For Health Professionals.* https://www.canada.ca/en/public-health/services/diseases/poliomyelitis-polio/health-professionals.html

Government of Canada. (2016, September 1). *Poliomyelitis vaccine: Canadian Immunization guide.* https://www.canada.ca/en/public-health/services/publications/healthy-living/canadian-immunization-guide-part-4-active-vaccines/page-17-poliomyelitis-vaccine.html

Greenwood, B. (2014). The contribution of vaccination to global health: Past, present and future. *Philosophical Transactions of the Royal Society B: Biological Sciences, 369*(1645), 20130433. https://doi.org/10.1098/rstb.2013.0433

Griffin, P. (2020, August 27). Explaining vaccine clinical trial phases. Retrieved May 17, 2021, from medicalxpress.com website: https://medicalxpress.com/news/2020-08-vaccine-clinical-trial-phases.html

Gruba, M. (2021, March 30). What happens if you get COVID after the first vaccine dose? Retrieved July 16, 2021, from RochesterFirst website: https://www.rochesterfirst.com/coronavirus/what-happens-if-you-get-covid-after-the-first-vaccine-dose/

Hamza, A., Wei, N. N., & Zhan, C. G. (2013). Ligand-based virtual screening approach using a new scoring function. National Institute of Health, 52(4), 963-974. doi:10.1021/ci200617d

HarperCollins Publishers. (n.d.). Tartaric acid. In *Collins English Dictionary*. Retrieved May 28, 2021, from https://www.collinsdictionary.com/dictionary/english/tararic-acid

Hawryluk, M., Kaiser Health News. (2021). Rural Americans in pharmacy deserts hurting for Covid-19 vaccines. Retrieved June 20, 2021 from https://www.cnn.com/2021/03/02/health/rural-pharmacy-deserts-covid-vaccines-khn/index.html

Hensley, L. (2020, December 23). What's the difference between a DNA and RNA Vaccine? Verywell Health. https://www.verywellhealth.com/ma-vs-dna-vaccine-5082285

Hilleman Film Team. (2019, October 28). *About Dr. Hilleman.* The Children's Hospital of Philadelphia. https://hillemanfilm.com/dr-hilleman

History.com Editors. (2021, May 30). Dr. Jonas Salk announces polio vaccine. *A&E Television Networks.* https://www.history.com/this-day-in-history/salk-announces-polio-vaccine

The History of Syphilis. (2017, July 27). Retrieved June 24, 2021, from STDAware Blog website: https://www.stdaware.com/blog/the-history-of-syphilis/

The History of Vaccines. (2018, January 10). Ethical Issues and Vaccines | History of Vaccines. Retrieved June 18, 2021, from Historyofvaccines.org website:

Hossain, K., Hassanzadeganroudsari, M., Apostolopoulos, V. (2021). The emergence of new strains of SARS-CoV-2. What does it mean for COVID-19 vaccines?, Expert Review of Vaccines, DOI: 10.1080/14760584.2021.1915140

HT Correspondent. (2021, July 2). *What is ZyCov-D, world's first DNA vaccine for COVID?* Hindustan Times. https://www.hindustantimes.com/india-news/what-is-zycov-d-world-s-first-dna-vaccine-for-covid-101625162617692.html

Huang, C., Huang, L., Wang, Y., Li, Xia., Ren, L., Gu, X., Kang, L., ...Cao, B. (2021). 6-month consequences of COVID-19 in patients discharged from hospital: a cohort study, The Lancet, (397)10270, 220-232, DOI:https://doi.org/10.1016/S0140-6736(20)32656-8

Huzar, T. (2020, October 26). Study identifies 3 existing drugs that may help treat COVID-19. *Medical News Today.* https://www.medicalnewstoday.com/articles/study-identifies-3-existing-drugs-that-may-help-treat-covid-19

Illinois Office of the Vice Chancellor for Research & Innovation. (n.d.). *Preventing Zoonotic Diseases.* https://research.illinois.edu/regulatory-compliance-safety/preventing-zoonotic-diseases

Institute of Medicine (US) Committee on the Evaluation of Vaccine Purchase Financing in the United States (2003). Vaccine Supply. Financing Vaccines in the 21st Century: Assuring Access and Availability. *National Academies Press (US).* https://www.ncbi.nlm.nih.gov/books/NBK221811/

Islam, M. S., Kamal, A. M., Kabir, A., Southern, D. L., Khan, S. H., Hasan, S., Sarkar, T., Sharmin, S., Das, S., Roy, T., Harun, M., Chughtai, A. A., Homaira, N., & Seale, H. (2021). COVID-19 vaccine rumors and conspiracy theories: The need for cognitive inoculation against misinformation to improve vaccine adherence. PloS one, 16(5), e0251605. https://doi.org/10.1371/journal.pone.0251605

Iwasaki, A., & Omer, S. B. (2020). Why and How Vaccines Work. *Cell, 183*(2), 290–295. https://doi.org/10.1016/j.cell.2020.09.040

Jain U. (2020). Effect of COVID-19 on the Organs. Cureus, 12(8), e9540. https://doi.org/10.7759/cureus.9540

Jang, Y. H., & Seong, B.-L. (2012). Principles underlying rational design of live attenuated influenza vaccines. *Clinical and Experimental Vaccine Research, 1*(1), 35–49. https://doi.org/10.7774/cevr.2012.1.1.35

Jean, S., Lee, P., Hsueh, P. (2020). Treatment options for COVID-19: The reality and challenges, Journal of Microbiology, Immunology and Infection, 53(3), 436-443. https://doi.org/10.1016/j.jmii.2020.03.034

Jean-Jacques, M., Bauchner, H. (2021). Vaccine Distribution— Equity Left Behind? JAMA, 325(9), 829–830. doi:10.1001/jama.2021.1205

Jia, W., Channappanavar, R., Zhang, C., Li, M., Zhou, H., Zhang, S., Zhou, P., Xu, J., Shan, S., Shi, X., Wang, X., Zhao, J., Zhou, D., Perlman, S., & Zhang, L. (2019). Single intranasal immunization with chimpanzee adenovirus-based vaccine induces sustained and protective immunity against MERS-CoV infection. Emerging microbes & infections, 8(1), 760–772. https://doi.org/10.1080/22221751.2019.1620083

Jimenez, D. (2021). Covid-19 vaccines: the role of social media in disinformation. Retrieved July 13, 2021 from https://www. pharmaceutical-technology.com/features/covid-19-vaccine-disinformation-social-media/

Johnson, S. (2018, September 17). Polio. *Healthline Media.* https://www.healthline.com/health/poliomyelitis

Kean, S. (2021, January 12). 22 orphans gave up everything to distribute the world's first vaccine. *The Atlantic.* https:// www.theatlantic.com/science/archive/2021/01/orphans-smallpox-vaccine-distribution/617646/

Kim, T. H., Johnstone, J., & Loeb, M. (2011). Vaccine herd effect. *Scandinavian Journal of Infectious Diseases, 43*(9), 683–689. https://doi.org/10.3109/00365548.2011.582247

King, L. S. (2021, May 13). Edward Jenner. In *Encyclopaedia Britannica.* Retrieved May 18, from https://www.britannica. com/biography/Edward-Jenner

Kommoss, F., Schwab, C., Tavernar, L., Schreck, J., Wagner, W. L., Merle, U., Jonigk, D., Schirmacher, P., & Longerich, T. (2020). The Pathology of Severe COVID-19-Related Lung Damage. Deutsches Arzteblatt international, 117(29-30), 500–506. https://doi.org/10.3238/arztebl.2020.0500

Kong, H. (2021, January 9). *What is the economic cost of COVID-19?* The Economist. https://www.economist.com/finance-and-economics/2021/01/09/what-is-the-economic-cost-of-covid-19

Krakow, M. (2019). *A tourist infected with measles visited Disneyland and other Southern California hot spots in mid-August.* Washington Post. https://www.washingtonpost.com/health/2019/08/24/tourist-infected-with-measles-visited-disneyland-other-southern-california-hotspots-mid-august/

Lam, S., Lombardi, A., & Ouanounou, A. (2020). COVID-19: A review of the proposed pharmacological treatments. European journal of pharmacology, 886, 173451. https://doi.org/10.1016/j.ejphar.2020.173451

Lauring, A. S., Hodcroft, E. B. (2021). Genetic Variants of SARS-CoV-2—What Do They Mean? JAMA. 325(6), 529–531. doi:10.1001/jama.2020.27124

Learn About Clinical Studies - ClinicalTrials.gov. (2019, March). Retrieved May 18, 2021, from U.S. National Library of Medicine website: https://clinicaltrials.gov/ct2/about-studies/learn

Leonhardt, D. (2021). The Vaccine Class Gap. Retrieved June 20, 2021 from https://www.nytimes.com/2021/05/24/briefing/vaccination-class-gap-us.html

Lewandowsky, S., Oberauer, K., & Gignac, G. E. (2013). NASA faked the moon landing—Therefore, (climate) science is a hoax: An anatomy of the motivated rejection of science. Psychological Science, 24, 622–633

Llamas, M. (2020, July 22). *Zithromax.* Drugwatch. https://www.drugwatch.com/zithromax-z-pak/

Lopez-Leon, S., Wegman-Ostrosky, T., Perelman, C., Sepulveda, R., Rebolledo, P. A., Cuapio, A., Villapol, S. (2021). More than 50 Long-term effects of COVID-19: a systematic review and meta-analysis, medRxiv, doi: https://doi.org/10.1101/2021.01.27.21250617.

Lord, J. M. (2013). The effect of aging of the immune system on vaccination responses, Human Vaccines & Immunotherapeutics, 9(6), 1364-1367, DOI: 10.4161/hv.24696

Lotfi, M., Hamblin, M. R., & Rezaei, N. (2020). COVID-19: Transmission, prevention, and potential therapeutic opportunities. Clinica chimica acta; international journal of clinical chemistry, 508, 254–266. https://doi.org/10.1016/j.cca.2020.05.044

MacArthur, A. C., McBride, M. L., Spinelli, J. J., Tamaro, S., Gallagher, R. P., Theriault, G. P. (2008). Risk of Childhood Leukemia Associated with Vaccination, Infection, and Medication Use in Childhood: The Cross-Canada Childhood Leukemia Study, American Journal of Epidemiology, 167(5), 598–606, https://doi.org/10.1093/aje/kwm339

Mackenzie, J. S., & Smith, D. W. (2020). COVID-19-A Novel Zoonotic Disease: A Review of the Disease, the Virus, and Public Health Measures. Asia-Pacific journal of public health, 32(4), 145–153. https://doi.org/10.1177/1010539520931326

Mallapaty, S. (2021). China COVID vaccine reports mixed results — what does that mean for the pandemic? Retrieved June 5, 2021 from https://www.nature.com/articles/d41586-021-00094-z

Markel, H. (2015, May 15). In 1850, Ignaz Semmelweus saved lives with three words: wash your hands. *PBS News Hour.* https://www.pbs.org/newshour/health/ignaz-semmelweis-doctor-prescribed-hand-washing

Mascola, J. R., Graham, B. S., Fauci, A. S. (2021). SARS-CoV-2 Viral Variants—Tackling a Moving Target. JAMA. 325(13), 1261–1262. doi:10.1001/jama.2021.2088

Mason, R. J. (2020). Pathogenesis of COVID-19 from a cell biology perspective, European Respiratory Journal, 55, DOI: 10.1183/13993003.00607-2020

Martin, D. (2018, July 9). Dr. Thomas Peebles – measles researcher – dies. New York Times. https://www.sfgate.com/bayarea/article/Dr-Thomas-Peebles-measles-researcher-dies-3179118.php

Maugh, T. (2005, April 13). *Maurice R. Hilleman, 85; Scientists developed many vaccines that saved millions of lives.* Los Angeles Times. https://www.latimes.com/archives/la-xpm-2005 -apr-13-me-hilleman13-story.html

Mayo Clinic. (2019, September 14). Anaphylaxis - Symptoms and causes. Retrieved July 8, 2021, from Mayo Clinic website: https://www.mayoclinic.org/diseases-conditions/anaphylaxis/symptoms-causes/syc-20351468

Mayo Clinic. (2020, September 22). Smallpox. https://www.mayoclinic.org/diseases-conditions/smallpox/symptoms-causes/syc-20353027

McRae, M. (2018, June 13). The Centuries of Not Having a Vaccine For Syphilis Could Finally Come to an End. Retrieved July 7, 2021, from ScienceAlert website: https://www.sciencealert.com/treponema-pallidum-syphilis-surface-marker-discovery-new-vaccine

Merriam-Webster. (n.d.). Endemic. In *Merriam-Webster. com dictionary.* Retrieved May 15, 2021, from https://www.merriam-webster.com/thesaurus/endemic

Merriam-Webster. (n.d.). Influenza. In *Merriam-Webster. com dictionary.* Retrieved June 6, 2021, from https://www.merriam-webster.com/dictionary/influenza

Merriam-Webster. (n.d.). 'Vaccine': The world's history ain't pretty. In *Merriam-Webster.com word history.* Retrieved May 20, 2021, from https://www.merriam-webster.com/words-at-play/vaccine-the-words-history-aint-pretty

Mocchegiani, E., Costarelli, L., Giacconi, R., Cipriano, C., Muti, E., & Malavolta, M. (2006). Zinc-binding proteins (metallothionein and alpha-2 macroglobulin) and immunosenescence. Experimental gerontology, 41(11), 1094–1107. https://doi.org/10.1016/j.exger.2006.08.010

Moore, S. (2021). What are adjuvants? News-Medical.Net. https://www.news-medical.net/life-sciences/What-are-Adjuvants.aspx

Mueller, A. L., McNamara, M. S., & Sinclair, D. A. (2020). Why does COVID-19 disproportionately affect older people?. Aging, 12(10), 9959–9981. https://doi.org/10.18632/aging.103344 Myocarditis Foundation. (n.d.). Discover Myocarditis Causes, Symptoms, Diagnosis, and Treatment. Retrieved May 22, 2021 from: https://www.myocarditisfoundation.org/about-myocarditis/.

Nascimento, I. P., & Leite, L. C. C. (2012). Recombinant vaccines and the development of new vaccine strategies. *Brazilian Journal of Medical and Biological Research, 45*(12), 1102–1111. https://doi.org/10.1590/S0100-879X2012007500142

National Center for Biotechnology Information. (2021). *Compound summary: Zuclopenthixol.* National Library of Medicine. https://pubchem.ncbi.nlm.nih.gov/compound/Zuclopenthixol

National Institutes of Health. (2021). Therapeutic Management of Adults With COVID-19. Retrieved May 23, 2021 from: https://www.covid19treatmentguidelines.nih.gov/therapeutic-management/.

National Institute on Alcohol Abuse and Alcoholism. (2020, May 12). *Drinking alcohol does not prevent or treat coronavirus infection and may impair immune function.* https://www.niaaa.nih.gov/news-events/announcement/drinking-alcohol-does-not-prevent-or-treat-coronavirus-infection-and-may-impair-immune-function

Ngan, V. (2008). *Cowpox.* DermNet NZ. https://dermnetnz.org/topics/cowpox/

Nix, E. (2019, July 29). Tuskegee Experiment: The Infamous Syphilis Study. Retrieved July 2, 2021, from HISTORY website: https://www.history.com/news/the-infamous-40-year-tuskegee-study

Novavax. (n.d.). Who is Novavax? Retrieved June 19, 2021 from https://www.novavax.com/about-us

Nuscheler, R. (2005). Monopoly Pricing in the Market for Vaccines. In On Competition and Regulation in Health Care Systems (NED-New edition, pp. 43–60). Peter Lang AG. http://www.jstor.org/stable/j.ctv9hj6kj.5

O'Donnell, C. (2021). Moderna booster increases antibodies against COVID-19 variants, early data shows. Retrieved June 27, 2021 from https://www.ctvnews.ca/health/coronavirus/moderna-booster-increases-antibodies-against-covid-19-variants-early-data-shows-1.5415554

Office of the Commissioner. (2019). Basics About Clinical Trials. Retrieved May 18, 2021, from U.S. Food and Drug Administration website: https://www.fda.gov/patients/clinical-trials-what-patients-need-know/basics-about-clinical-trials

Office of Infectious Disease and HIV/AIDS Policy. (2021, April 29). Vaccine types. Health and Human Services Government. https://www.hhs.gov/immunization/basic/types/index.html

Oliveira, D. S., Medeiros, N. I., & Gomes, J. (2020). Immune response in COVID-19: What do we currently know?. Microbial pathogenesis, 148, 104484. https://doi.org/10.1016/j.micpath.2020.104484

Oliver, M. (2019, April 17). "You Don't Treat Dogs That Way": The Horrifying Story Of The Tuskegee Experiment. Retrieved June 30, 2021, from All That's Interesting website: https://allthatsinteresting.com/tuskegee-experiment-syphilis-study

Ontario Ministry of Health. (2021). Administration of AstraZeneca COVID-19 Vaccine/COVISHIELD Vaccine. Retrieved June 12, 2021 from https://www.health.gov.on.ca/en/pro/programs/publichealth/coronavirus/docs/vaccine/COVID-19_AstraZeneca_Vaccine_admin.pdf

Orkin. (2021). *Anopheles mosquito facts & identification: How to prevent and control anopheles mosquitoes.* https://www.orkin.com/other/mosquitoes/anopheles-mosquito

Østergaard, S. D., Schmidt, M., Horváth-Puhó, E., Thomsen, R. W., & Sørensen, H. T. (2021). Thromboembolism and the Oxford-AstraZeneca COVID-19 vaccine: side-effect or coincidence?. Lancet (London, England), 397(10283), 1441–1443. https://doi.org/10.1016/S0140-6736(21)00762-5

Ouassou, H., Kharchoufa, L., Bouhrim, M., Daoudi, N. E., Imtara, H., Bencheikh, N., ELbouzidi, A., Bnouham, M. (2020). "The Pathogenesis of Coronavirus Disease 2019 (COVID-19): Evaluation and Prevention", Journal of Immunology Research. https://doi.org/10.1155/2020/1357983

Oxford Vaccine Group. (n.d.). Vaccine Knowledge Project. Retrieved June 11, 2021 from https://vk.ovg.ox.ac.uk/vk/covid-19-vaccines

Pawelec, G., McElhaney, J. (2021). Unanticipated efficacy of SARS-CoV-2 vaccination in older adults. Immunity & Ageing, 18(7). https://doi.org/10.1186/s12979-021-00219-y

Pfizer. (n.d.). The Facts About the Pfizer-BioNTech COVID-19 Vaccine. Retrieved June 11, 2021 from https://www.pfizer.com/news/hot-topics/the_facts_about_pfizer_and_biontech_s_covid_19_vaccine

Plotkin, S., Robinson, J. M., Cunningham, G., Iqbal, R., & Larsen, S. (2017). The complexity and cost of vaccine manufacturing – An overview. Vaccine, 35(33), 4064–4071. https://doi.org/10.1016/j.vaccine.2017.06.003

Polack, F. P., Thomas, S. J., Kitchin, N., Absalon, J., Gurtman, A., Lockhart, S., Perez, J. L., Pérez Marc, G., Moreira, E. D., Zerbini, C., Bailey, R., Swanson, K. A., Roychoudhury, S., Koury, K., Li, P., Kalina, W. V., Cooper, D., Frenck, R. W., Jr, Hammitt, L. L., Türeci, Ö., ... C4591001 Clinical Trial Group (2020). Safety and Efficacy of the BNT162b2 mRNA Covid-19 Vaccine. The New England journal of medicine, 383(27), 2603–2615. https://doi.org/10.1056/NEJMoa2034577

Pollard, A. J., & Bijker, E. M. (2021). A guide to vaccinology: From basic principles to new developments. *Nature Reviews Immunology, 21*(2), 83–100. https://doi.org/10.1038/s41577-020-00479-7

Pouton, C. (2020, May 21). Explained: The challenges in developing a COVID-19 vaccine. Retrieved July 10, 2021, from Monash Lens website: https://lens.monash.edu/@coronavirus-articles/2020/05/21/1380490/explained-the-challenges-of-developing-a-covid-19-vaccine#

Prescription Medicines Code of Practice Authority. (2021). *What does the future of vaccines look like?* ABPI. https://www.abpi.org.uk/new-medicines/vaccines/the-future-of-vaccines/

Public Health Associations of BC. (2021). *Why your child needs to get vaccinated on time.* https://immunizebc.ca/why-your-child-needs-get-vaccinated-on-time

Public Health Agency of Canada. (2019). Vaccines for children: Vaccine safety, concerns and side effects - Canada.ca. Retrieved July 8, 2021, from Canada.ca website: https://www.canada.ca/en/public-health/services/vaccination-children/safety-concerns-side-effects.html

Public Health Ontario. (2020). COVID-19 – What We Know So Far About... Zoonotic Origins. Retrieved May 17, 2021 from: https://www.publichealthontario.ca/-/media/documents/ncov/what-we-know-feb-26-2020.pdf?la=en.

Pulendran, B., & Ahmed, R. (2011). Immunological mechanisms of vaccination. *Nature Immunology, 12*(6), 509–517.

Raivio K. (1990). Miten lapsikuolleisuus vaikuttaa syntyvyyteen? [How does infant mortality affect birth rates?]. Duodecim; laaketieteellinen aikakauskirja, 106(17), 1187–1189.

Randolph, H. E., & Barreiro, L. B. (2020). *Herd Immunity: Understanding COVID-19. Immunity, 52*(5), 737–741. https://doi.org/10.1016/j.immuni.2020.04.012

Richman D. D. (2021). COVID-19 vaccines: implementation, limitations and opportunities. Global health & medicine, 3(1), 1–5. https://doi.org/10.35772/ghm.2021.01010

Riedel, S. (2005). Edward Jenner and the history of smallpox and vaccination. *Baylor University Medical Center Proceedings, 18*(1), 21-25. https://dx.doi.org/10.1080%2F08998280.2005.11928028

Ries, J. (2021). *The Coronavirus Is Mutating: What to Know About New Variants.* Healthline. https://www.healthline.com/health-news/the-coronavirus-is-mutating-what-we-know-about-the-new-variants

Rogers, K. (2019). Guatemala syphilis experiment | American medical research project. In *Encyclopædia Britannica.* Retrieved from https://www.britannica.com/event/Guatemala-syphilis-experiment

Rogers, L. S., & Health, J. B. S. of P. (2021). *What is Herd Immunity and How Can We Achieve It With COVID-19?* Johns Hopkins Bloomberg School of Public Health. Retrieved July 19, 2021, from https://www.jhsph.edu/covid-19/articles/achieving-herd-immunity-with-covid19.html

Rouw, A., Kates, J., Michaud, J., Wexler, M. (2021). COVAX and the United States. Retrieved June 19, 2021 from https://www.kff.org/coronavirus-covid-19/issue-brief/covax-and-the-united-states/

Roux, A., Wexler, A., Kates, J., Michaud, J. (2021). Global COVID-19 Vaccine Access: A Snapshot of Inequality. Retrieved June 19, 2021 from https://www.kff.org/policy-watch/global-covid-19-vaccine-access-snapshot-of-inequality/

Ryan, L. (2021, February 2). What Does Vaccine Efficacy Rate Mean? Retrieved July 22, 2021, from ideastream website: https://www.ideastream.org/news/what-does-vaccine-efficacy-rate-mean

Sandhu, V. (2020, April). Hydroxychloroquine (Plaquenil). *American College of Rheumatology.* https://www.rheumatology.org/I-Am-A/Patient-Caregiver/Treatments/Hydroxychloroquine-Plaquenil

Santos, A. F., Gaspar, P. D., de Souza, H. J. L. (2021). Refrigeration of COVID-19 Vaccines: Ideal Storage Characteristics, Energy Efficiency and Environmental Impacts of Various Vaccine Options. Energies, 14(7), 1849. https://doi.org/10.3390/en14071849

Schenkelberg T. (2021). Vaccine-induced protection in aging adults and pandemic response. Biochemical and biophysical research communications, 538, 218–220. https://doi.org/10.1016/j.bbrc.2020.10.090

Science History Institute. (2021). *Jonas Salk and Alberta Bruce Sabin.* http://www.sciencehistory.org/historical-profile/jonas-salk-and-albert-bruce-sabin

Seladi-Schulman, J. (2021, March 5). Why Two Doses of COVID-19 Vaccine for Pfizer and Moderna? Retrieved July 20, 2021, from Healthline website: https://www.healthline.com/health/why-two-doses-of-covid-vaccine#why-two-doses

Shang, J., Ye, G., Shi, K., Wan, Y., Luo, C., Aihara, H., Geng, Q., Auerbach, A., & Li, F. (2020). Structural basis of receptor recognition by SARS-CoV-2. Nature, 581(7807), 221–224. https://doi.org/10.1038/s41586-020-2179-y

Sheldon, M. (2021, June 9). The difficulty of vaccinating the world against COVID-19 is enormous. Retrieved from CBC website: https://www.cbc.ca/news/world/global-vaccine-supply-1.6056550

Shepherd, K. (2020, March 24). *A man thought aquarium cleaner with the same name as the anti-viral drug chloroquine would prevent coronavirus. It killed him.* The Washington Post. https://www.washingtonpost.com/nation/2020/03/24/coronavirus-chloroquine-poisoning-death/

Sheridan, C. (2005). The business of making vaccines. *Nature Biotechnology, 23*(11), 1359. https://doi.org/10.1038/nbt1105-1359

Soiza, R. L., Scicluna, C., & Thomson, E. C. (2021). Efficacy and safety of COVID-19 vaccines in older people. Age and ageing, 50(2), 279–283. https://doi.org/10.1093/ageing/afaa274

Solana, R., Pawelec, G. (2004). Immunosenescence, NeuroImmune Biology, 4, 9-21. https://doi.org/10.1016/S1567-7443(04)80003-6.

Sommerfeldt, C. (2020, May 27). White House refuses to release letter from N.Y. doctor that Trump claims praised hydroxychloroquine. *New York Daily News.* https://www.nydailynews.com/coronavirus/ny-coronavirus-white-house-doctor-letter-trump-Hydroxychloroquine-20200527-wwk43jng25el3bwz63b4xupsty-story.html

Sriskandarajah, I. (2021). Where did the microchip vaccine conspiracy theory come from anyway?. Retrieved July 13, 2021 from https://revealnews.org/article/where-did-the-microchip-vaccine-conspiracy-theory-come-from-anyway/

Stein R. A. (2017). The golden age of anti-vaccine conspiracies. Germs, 7(4), 168–170. https://doi.org/10.18683/germs.2017.1122

Stewart, A. J., & Devlin, P. M. (2005). The history of the smallpox vaccine. *Journal of Infection, 52*(5), 329-334. https://doi.org/10.1016/j.jinf.2005.07.021

Stewart, M. (2018, July 27). *Zuclopenthixol: Clopixol.* Egton Medical Information Systems Limited. https://patient.info/medicine/zuclopenthixol-clopixol

Strauss, J. H., & Strauss E. J. (2008). DNA-containing viruses. *Viruses and Human Disease.* Retrieved June 9, 2021, from https://www.sciencedirect.com/topics/neuroscience/alastrim

Syphilis - Symptoms and causes. (2018). Retrieved June 23, 2021, from Mayo Clinic website: https://www.mayoclinic.org/diseases-conditions/syphilis/symptoms-causes/syc-20351756

Tellado, M. P. (2019, March). *Do my kids need vaccines before traveling?* The Nemours Foundation. https://kidshealth.org/en/parents/travel-vaccinations.html

Tikkanen, A. (n.d.). Cowpox. In *Encyclopedia Britannica.* Retrieved May 18, 2021, from https://www.britannica.com/science/cowpox

Tikkanen, A. (2021). Ramses V: King of Egypt. In *Encyclopedia Britannica.* Retrieved May 15, 2021, from https://britannica.com/biography/Ramses-V

Tulchinsky, T. H. (2018). Maurice Hilleman: Creator of vaccines that changed the world. *Elsevier Public Health Emergency Collection,* 443-470. https://dx.org/10.1016%2FB 978-0-12-804571-8.00003-2

Ullmann, A. (n.d). Louis Pasteur: French chemist and microbiologist. In *Encyclopedia Britannica.* Retrieved May 28, 2021, from https://www.britannica.com/biography/Louis-Pasteur

Ulmer, J. B., & Liu, M. (2021). Path to success and future impact of nucleic acid vaccines: DNA and mRNA. *Molecular Frontiers Journal, 5*(1), 1-20. doi:10.1142/S252973251400022

UPMC Center for Health Security. (2014, February 26). *Variola virus (smallpox).* Johns Hopkins University. https://www.centerforhealthsecurity.org/our-work/publications/smallpox-fact-sheet

U.S. Food & Drug Administration. (2020, November 20). Emergency use authorization for vaccines explained. FDA. https://www.fda.gov/vaccines-blood-biologics/vaccines/emergency-use-authorization-vaccines-explained

U.S. Food & Drug Administration. (n.d.). *Biological product definitions.* FDA. https://www.fda.gov/files/drugs/published/Biological-Product-Definitions.pdf

U.S. National Library of Medicine. (2017). *Amodiaquine.* LiverTox: Clinical and Research Information on Drug-Induced Liver Injury. https://www.ncbi.nlm.nih.gov/books/NBK548404/pdf/Bookshelf_NBK548404.pdf

U.S. National Library of Medicine. (2021, June 8). *Nebivolol.* MedlinePlus. https://medlineplus.gov/druginfo/meds/ a608029.html

Van Prooijen, J. W., & Douglas, K. M. (2017). Conspiracy theories as part of history: The role of societal crisis situations. Memory studies, 10(3), 323–333. https://doi. org/10.1177/1750698017701615

VBI Vaccines. (2016, November 23). *Louis Pasteur and the development of the attenuated vaccine.* https://www. vbivaccines.com/evlp-platform/louis-pasteur-attenuated-vaccine/

The Virality Project. (n.d.). Announcing the Virality Project. Retrieved July 13, 2021 from https://www.viralityproject.org/ news/about

Wadman, M. (2020). Will a small, long-shot U.S. company end up producing the best coronavirus vaccine?. Retrieved June 20, 2021 from https://www.sciencemag.org/news/2020/11/ will-small-long-shot-us-company-end-producing-best-coronavirus-vaccine

Wadman, M., Couzin-Frankel, J., Kaiser, J., Matacic, C. (2020). How does coronavirus kill? Clinicians trace a ferocious rampage through the body, from brain to toes, Science Mag. Retrieved May 17, 2021 from: https://www.sciencemag.org/ news/2020/04/how-does-coronavirus-kill-clinicians-trace-ferocious-rampage-through-body-brain-toes.

Walter, E. B., & Moody, M. A. (2021). Vaccine Development: Steps to Approval of an Investigational Vaccine. *North Carolina Medical Journal, 82*(2), 141–144. https://doi.org/10.18043/ncm.82.2.141

WebMD. (2021). Hydroxychloroquine. https://www.webmd.com/lung/hydroxychloroquine#1

Whaley, M. M., Byers-Connon, S., Lane, J., Carruthers, C., Walker, L., Lancaster D. B. (2019). Chapter 3 - The Aging Process, Occupational Therapy with Elders, 4, 30-40. https://doi.org/10.1016/B978-0-323-49846-3.00003-2.

Wiersinga W. J., Rhodes A., Cheng A. C., Peacock S. J., Prescott H. C. (2020). Pathophysiology, Transmission, Diagnosis, and Treatment of Coronavirus Disease 2019 (COVID-19): A Review.

JAMA, 324(8), 782–793. doi:10.1001/jama.2020.12839 Wong, M. C., Javornik Cregeen, S. J., Ajami, N. J., Petrosino, J. F. (2020). Evidence of recombination in coronaviruses implicating pangolin origins of nCoV-2019. https://doi.org/10.1101/2020.02.07.939207

World Health Organization. (2021). WHO Coronavirus (COVID-19) Dashboard. Retrieved May 15, 2021 from: https://covid19.who.int/.

World Health Organization. (2021, May 5). *Coronavirus disease (COVID-19) advice for the public: Mythbusters.* https://www.who.int/emergencies/diseases/novel-coronavirus-2019/advice-for-public/myth-busters#garlic

World Health Organization. (2021). Protect yourself and others from COVID-19. Retrieved May 21, 2021 from: https://www.who.int/emergencies/diseases/novel-coronavirus-2019/advice-for-public.

World Health Organization. (2020, April 27). *Archived: WHO timeline – COVID-19.* https://www.who.int/news/item/27-04-2020-who-timeline---covid-19

World Health Organization. (2020). *Coronavirus disease (COVID-19): Vaccines.* Retrieved June 27 from https://www.who.int/news-room/q-a-detail/coronavirus-disease-(covid-19)-vaccines,

World Health Organization. (2020). *Global Vaccine Market Report.* https://www.who.int/immunization/programmes_systems/procurement/mi4a/platform/module2/2020_Global_Vaccine_Market_Report.pdf?ua=1

World Health Organization. (2020). *Vaccines and immunization: What is vaccination?* https://www.who.int/news-room/q-a-detail/vaccines-and-immunization-what-is-vaccination?

World Health Organization. (2019, December 5). *Measles.* https://www.who.int/news-room/fact-sheets/detail/measles

World Health Organization. (2019, June 14). *Sanitation.* https://www.who.int/news-room/fact-sheets/detail/sanitation

Worldometer. (2021, July 8). *COVID-19 coronavirus pandemic [Weekly trends].* Retrieved July 8, 2021, from https://www.worldometers.info/coronavirus/?utm_campaign=homeAdUOA?Si

Wu, Z., Hu, Y., Xu, M., Chen, Z., Yang, W., Jiang, Z., Li, M., ...Yin, W. (2021). Safety, tolerability, and immunogenicity of an inactivated SARS-CoV-2 vaccine (CoronaVac) in healthy adults aged 60 years and older: a randomised, double-blind, placebo-controlled, phase 1/2 clinical trial, The Lancet, Infectious Diseases, (21)6, 803-812, DOI:https://doi.org/10.1016/S1473-3099(20)30987-7

Yelin, D., Wirtheim, E., Vetter, P., Kalil, A. C., Bruchfeld, J., Runold, M., Guaraldi, G., Mussini, C., Gudiol, C., Pujol, M., Bandera, A., Scudeller, L., Paul, M., Kaiser, L., & Leibovici, L. (2020). Long-term consequences of COVID-19: research needs. The Lancet. Infectious diseases, 20(10), 1115–1117. https://doi.org/10.1016/S1473-3099(20)30701-5

Zhang, L., Wang, W., & Wang, S. (2015). Effect of vaccine administration modality on immunogenicity and efficacy. Expert review of vaccines, 14(11), 1509–1523. https://doi.org/10.1586/14760584.2015.1081067

Zhang, S. (2015, August 4). The U.S. Doctor Who Infected 1,300 Guatemalan Patients With STDs. Retrieved July 3, 2021, from Gizmodo website: https://gizmodo.com/the-u-s-doctor-who-infected-1-300-guatemalan-patients-1696095744

www.ingramcontent.com/pod-product-compliance
Lightning Source LLC
Chambersburg PA
CBHW071740270326
41928CB00013B/2751